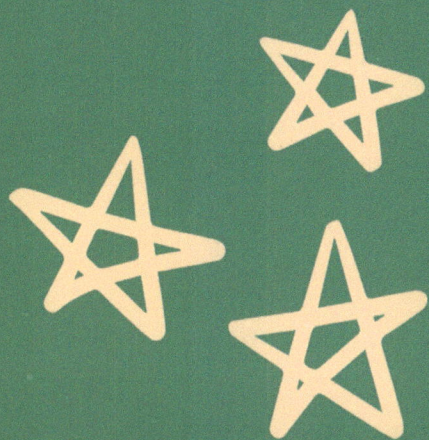

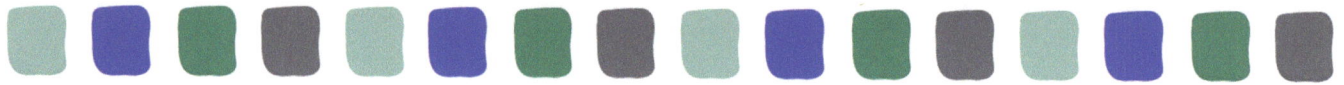

This book is dedicated to:

My two beautiful children, JJ and Jade
and
girls and boys that are excited to learn how to stay focused,
understand how you feel, and improve your well-being
while you are in and out of school.

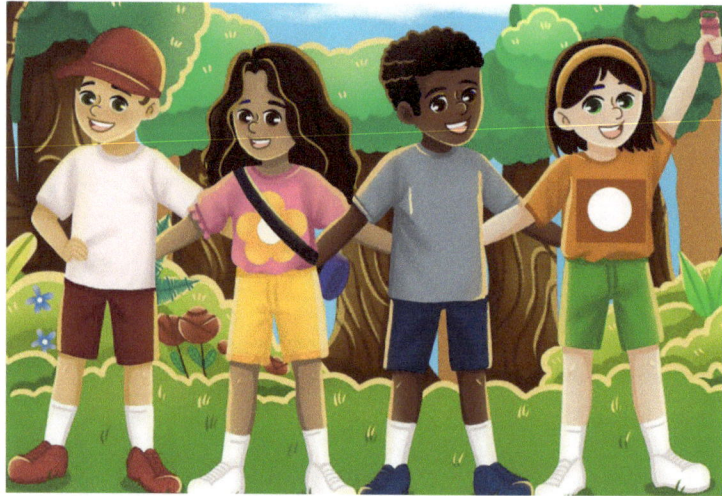

Copyright 2023 by Ashleigh Abney.

For more books, visit us online at
empowerbooksforkids.net

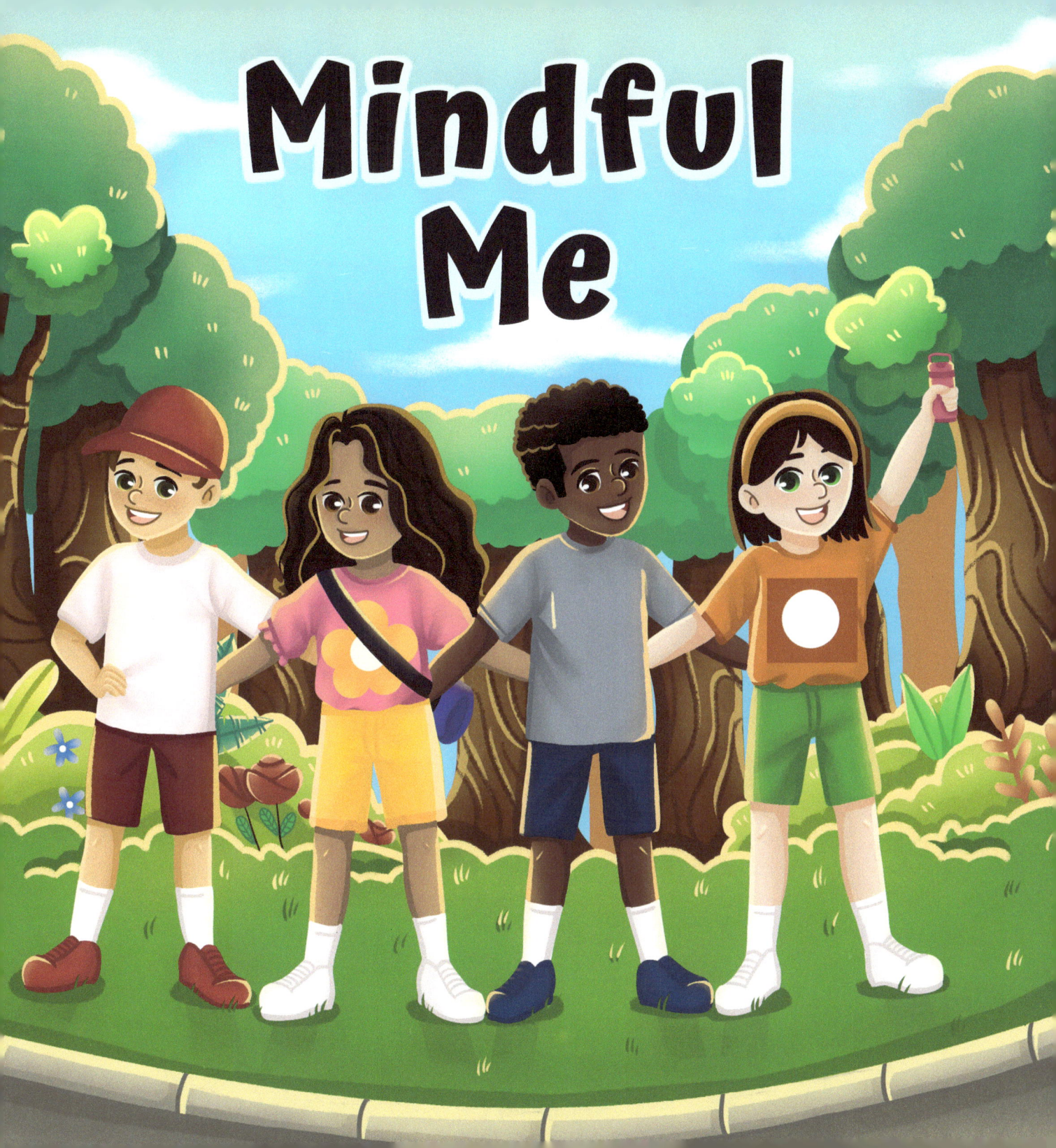

Mindful Me

In a world so big and loud,

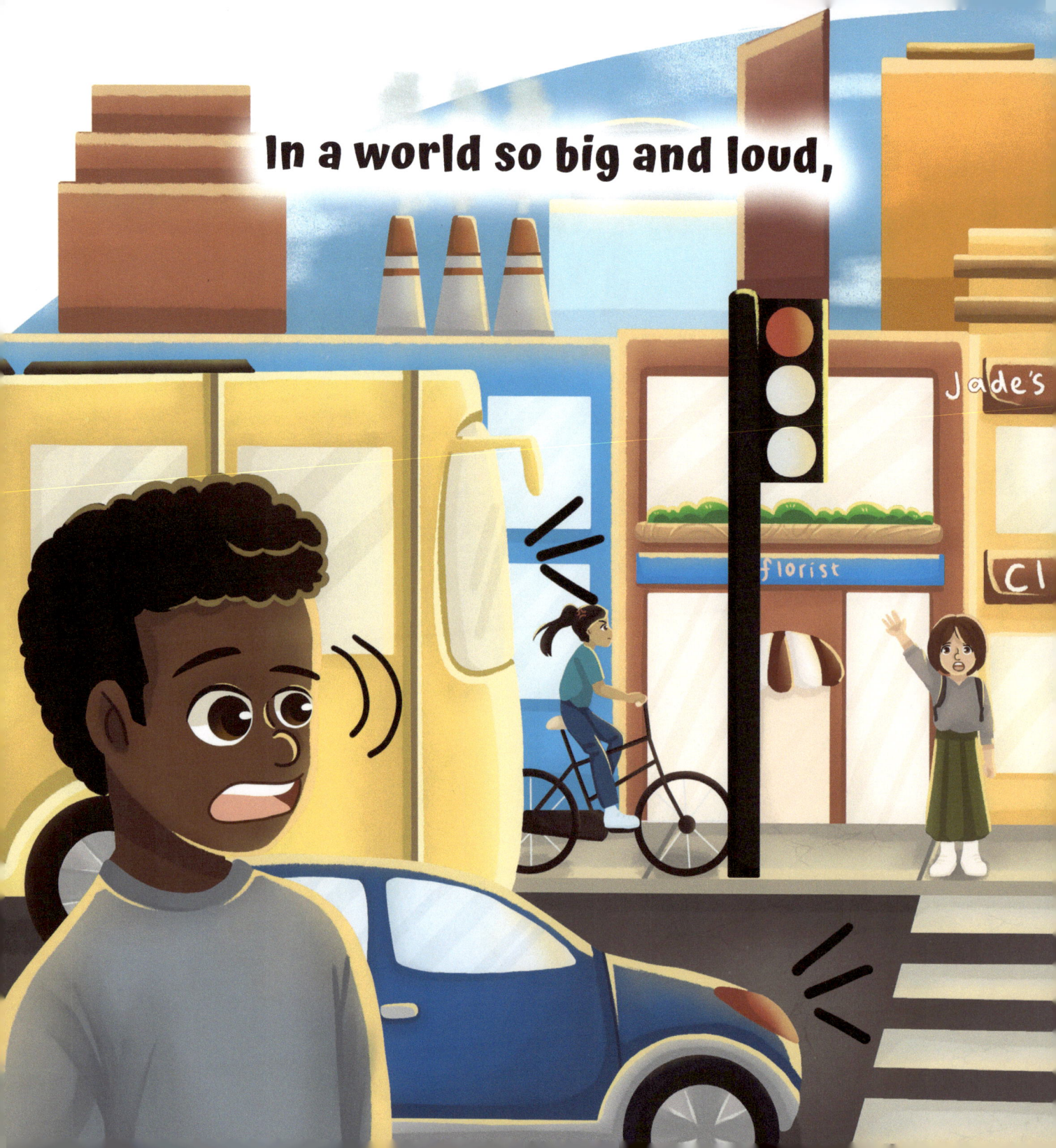

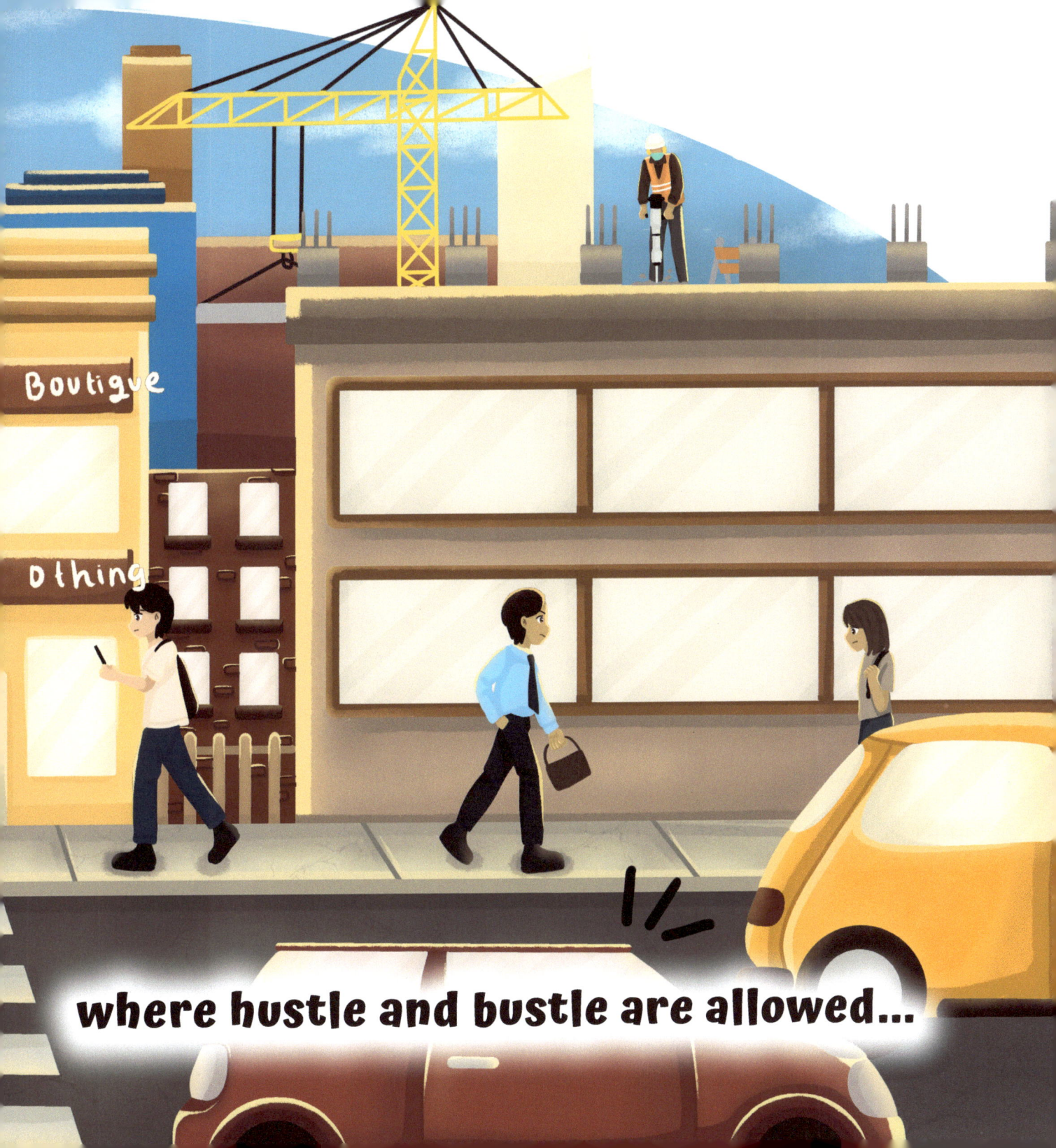

where hustle and bustle are allowed...

There is a magic key to find,

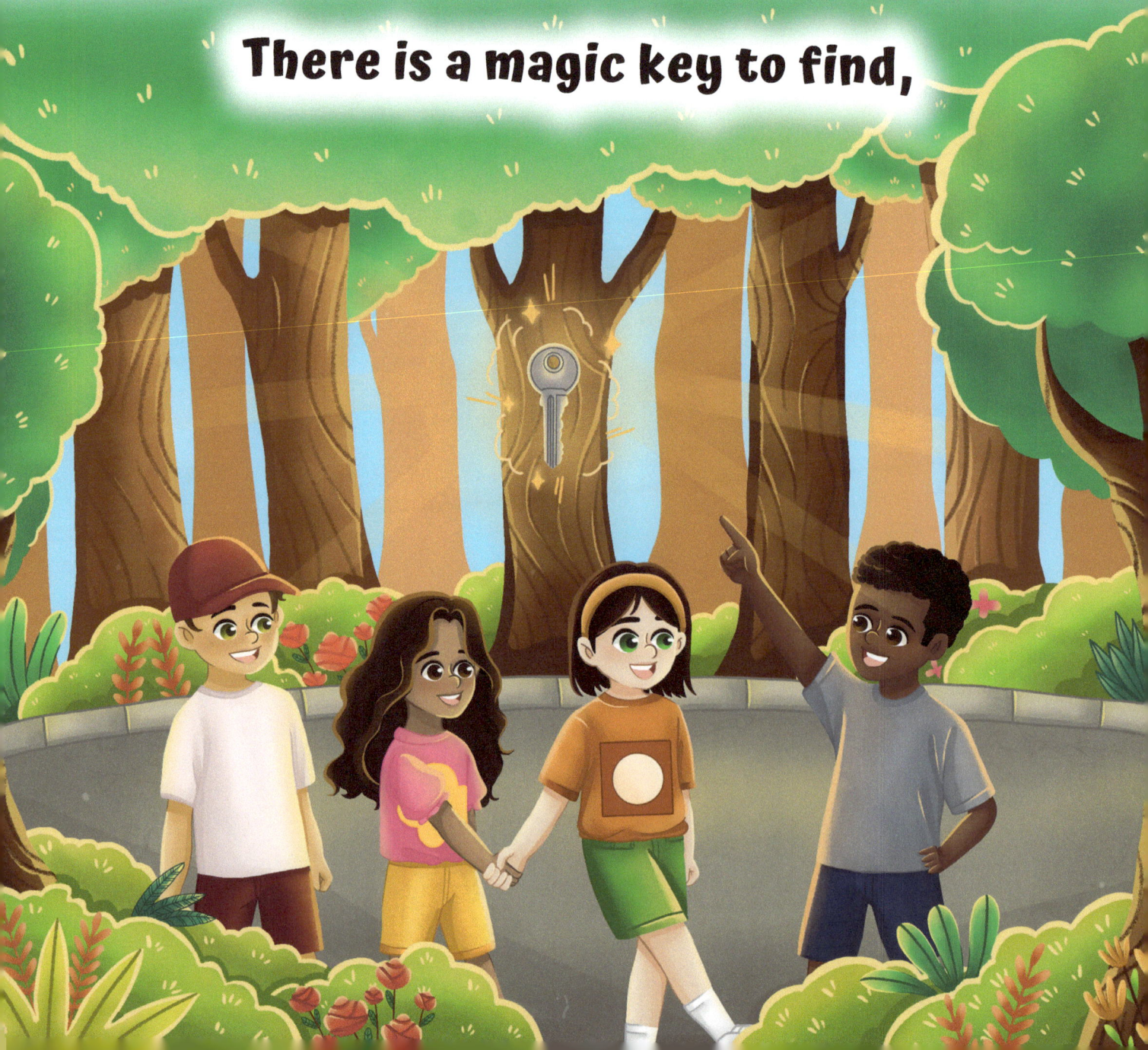

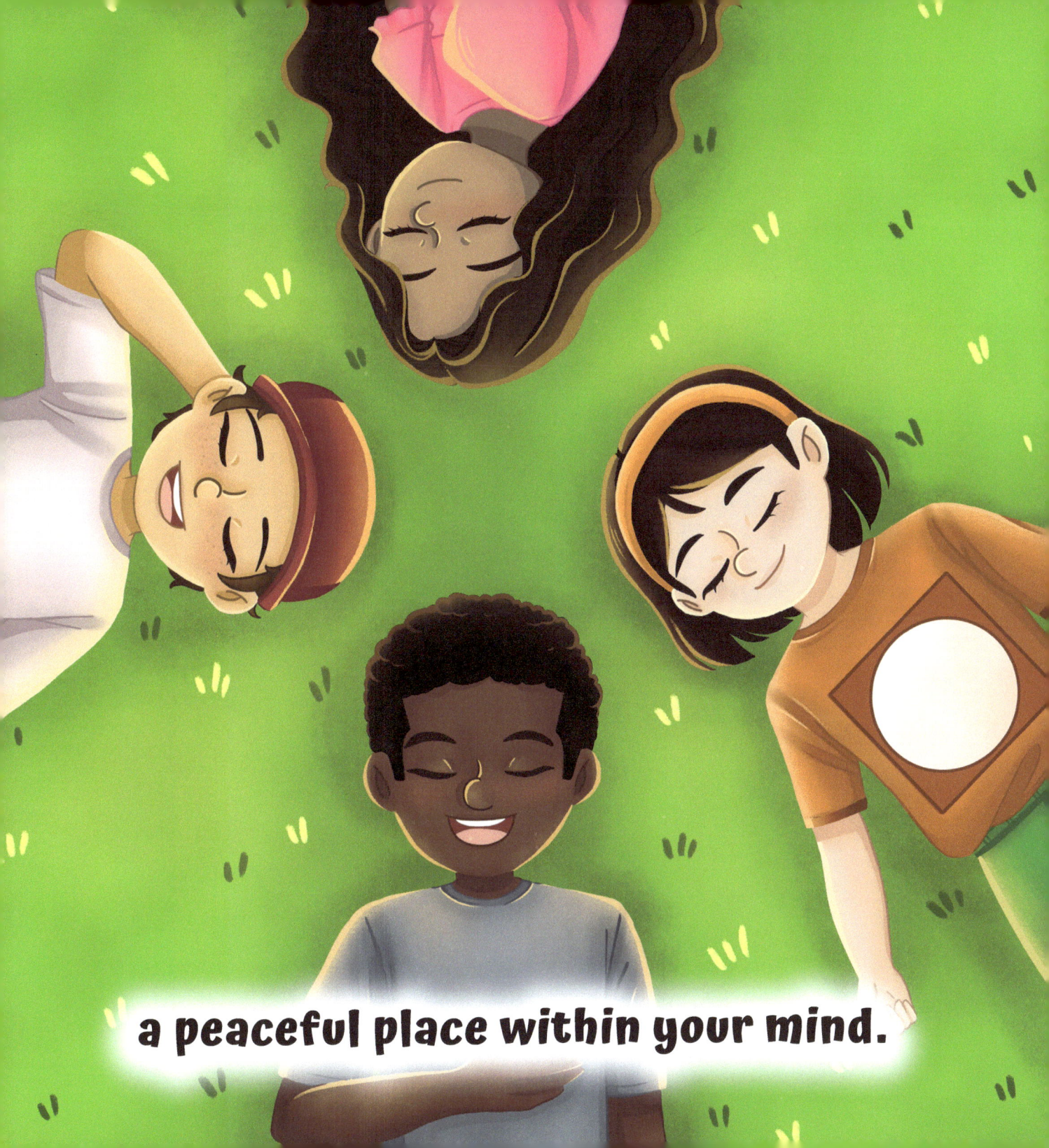

a peaceful place within your mind.

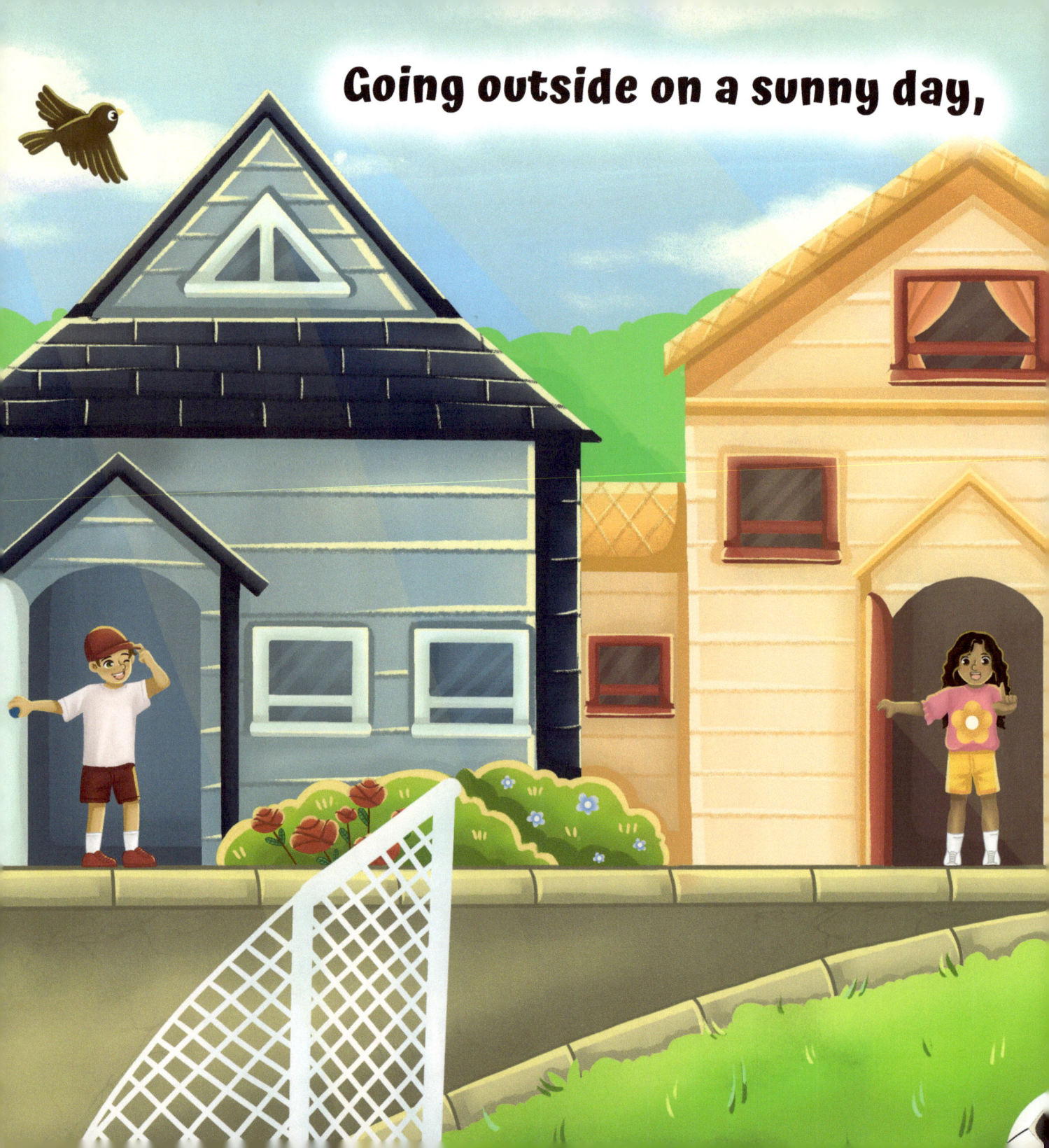

Going outside on a sunny day,

can bring us joy when it's time to play.

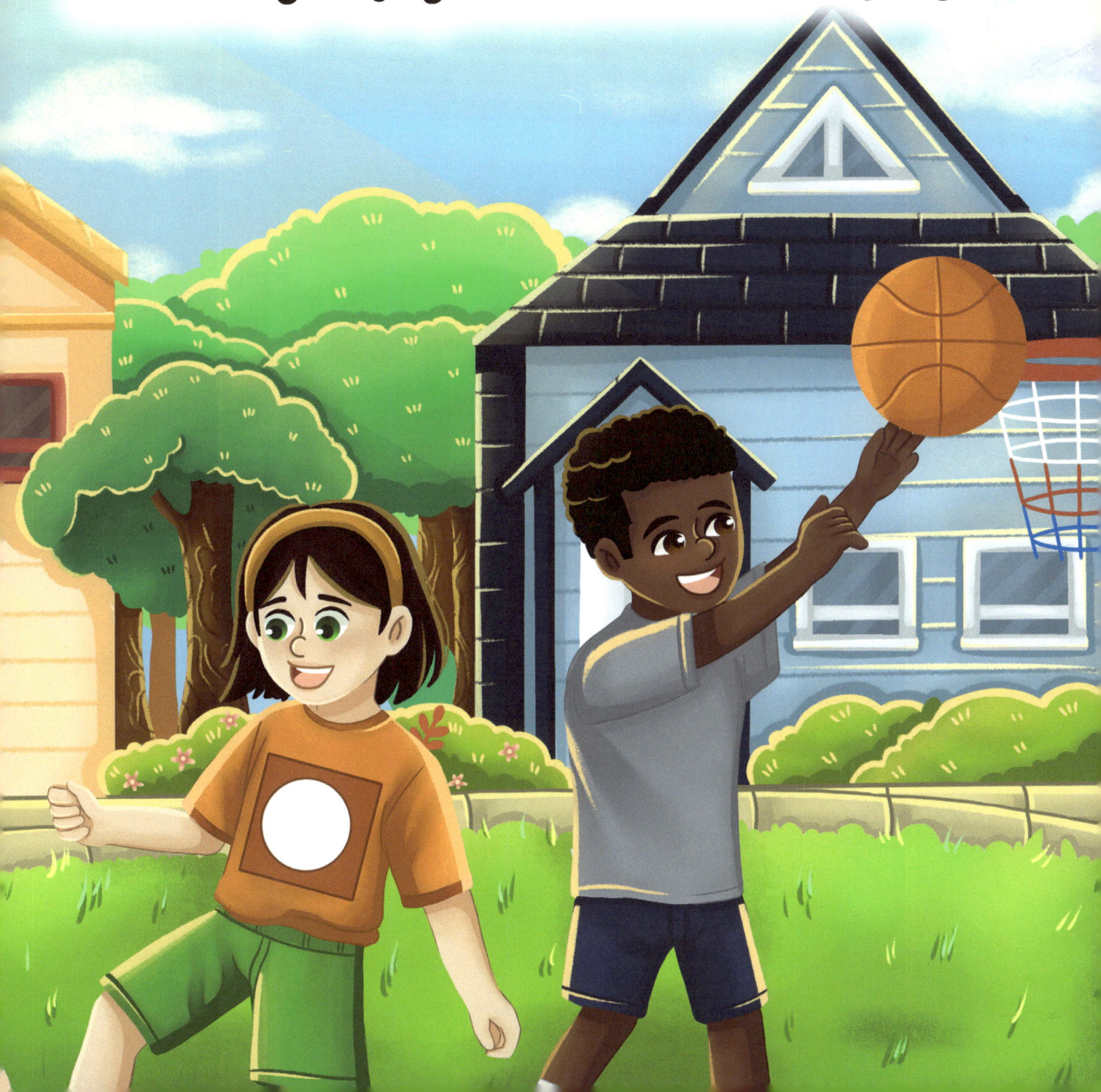

You can ride a bike or go for a walk,

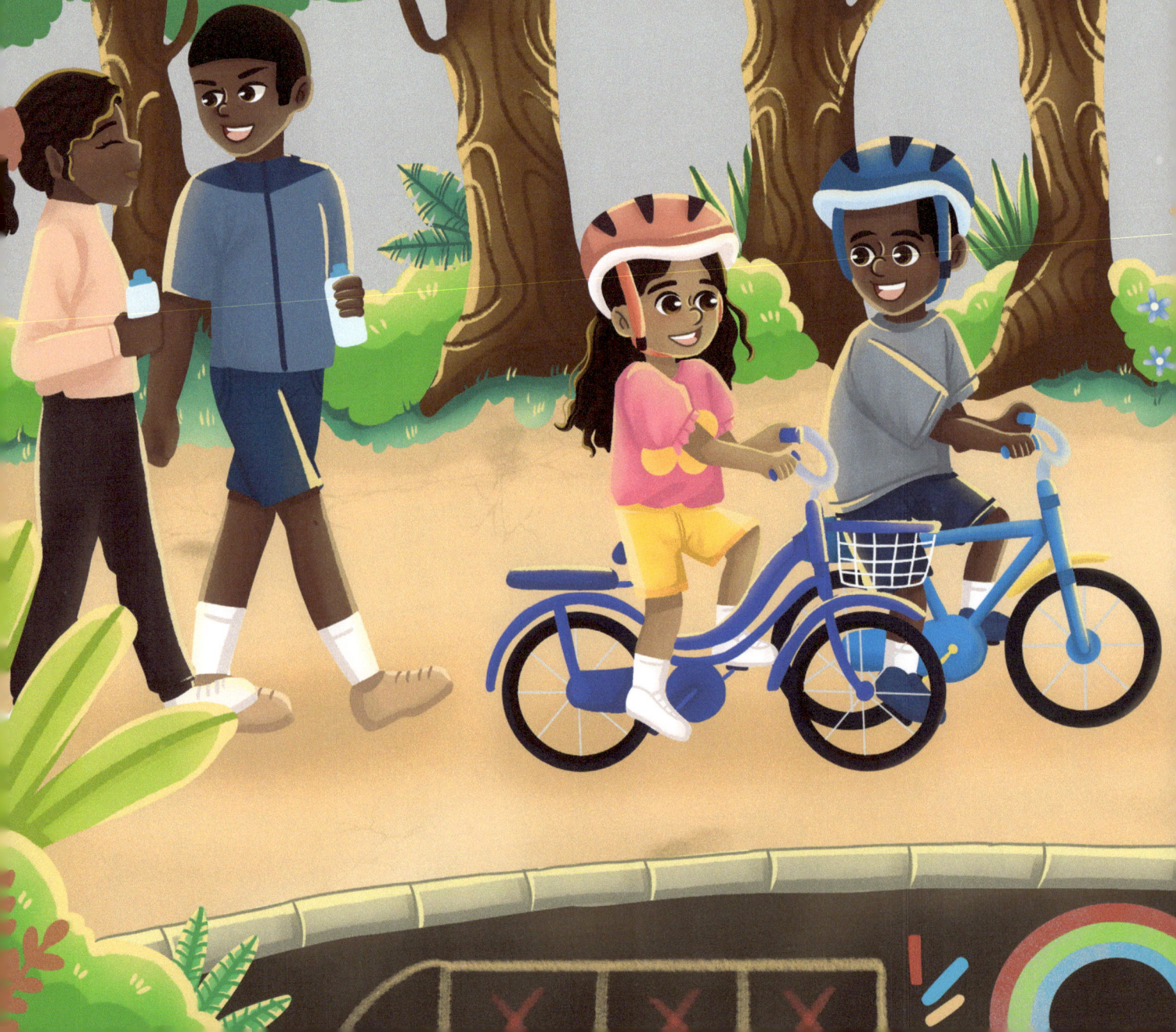

you can check out nature or
draw with chalk.

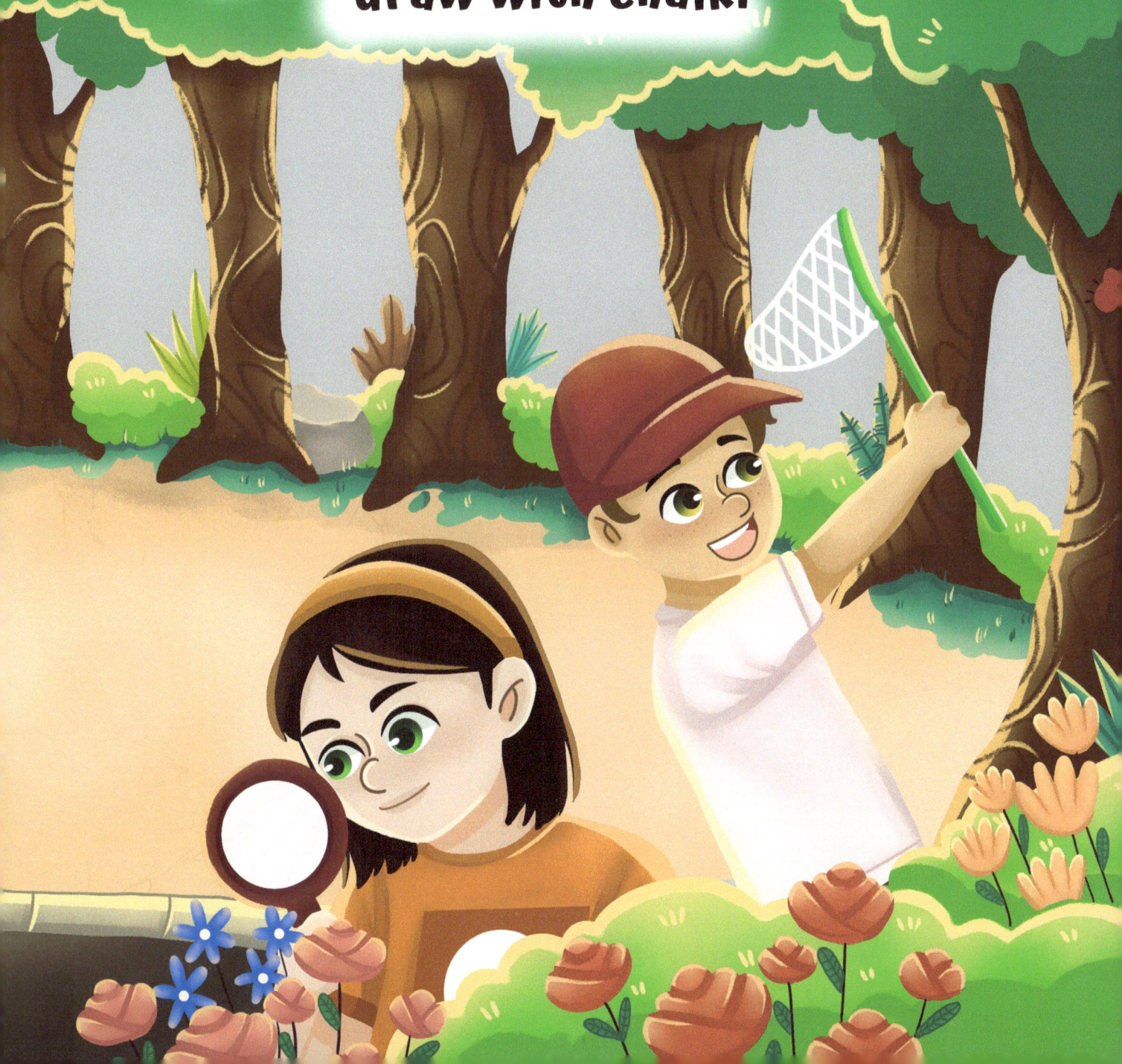

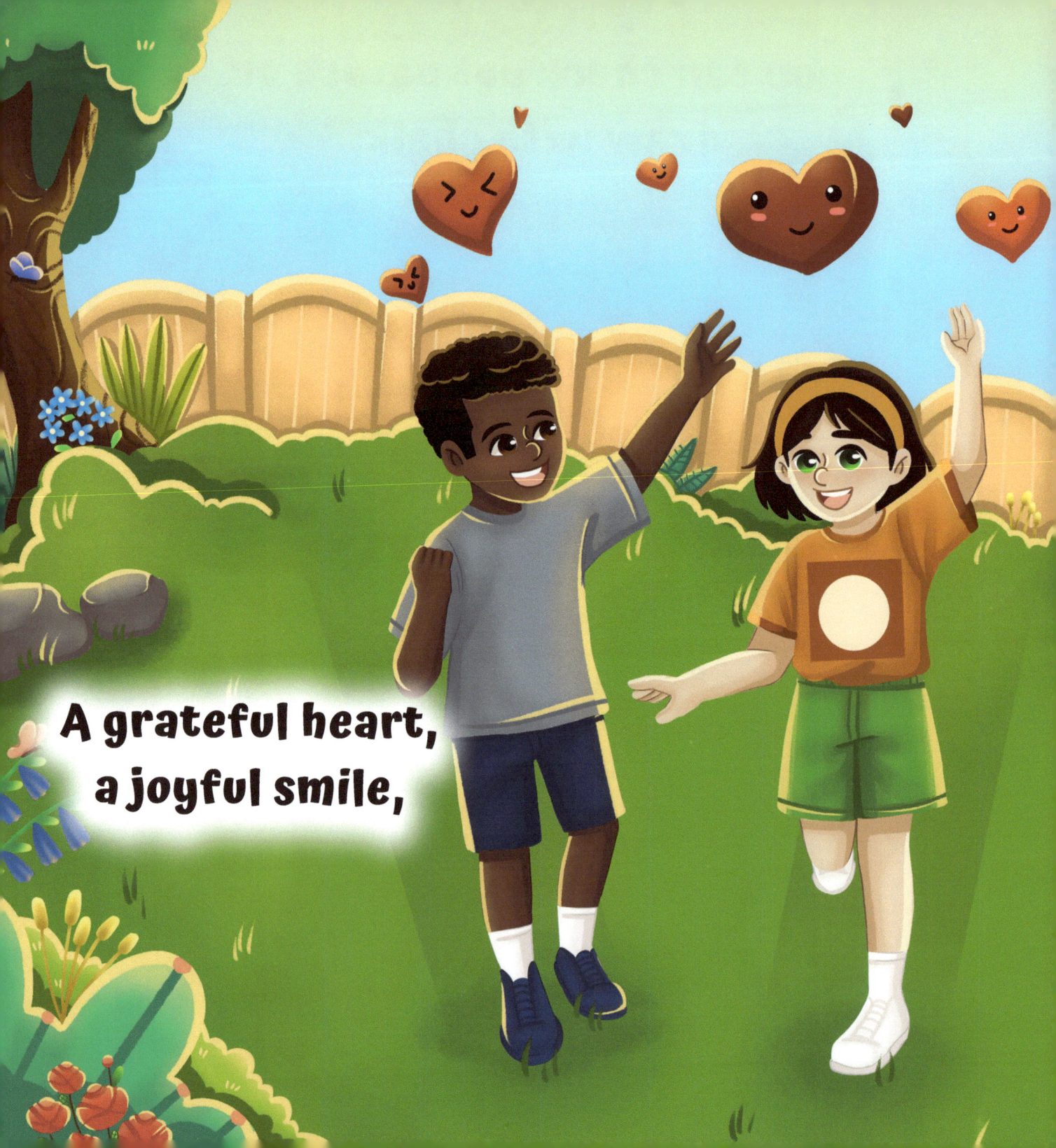

A grateful heart,
a joyful smile,

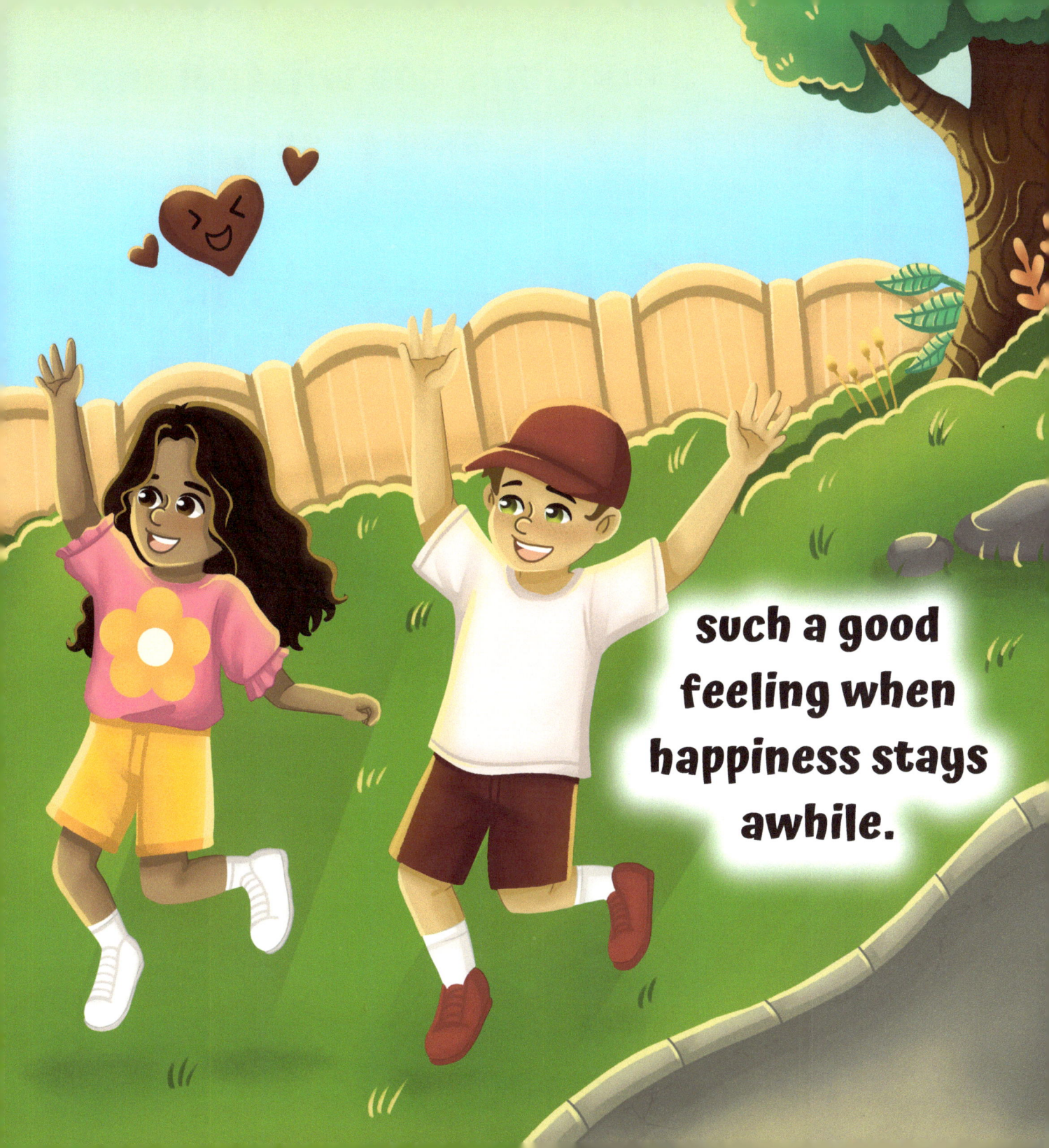

such a good
feeling when
happiness stays
awhile.

Sometimes you will feel angry, mad or sad,

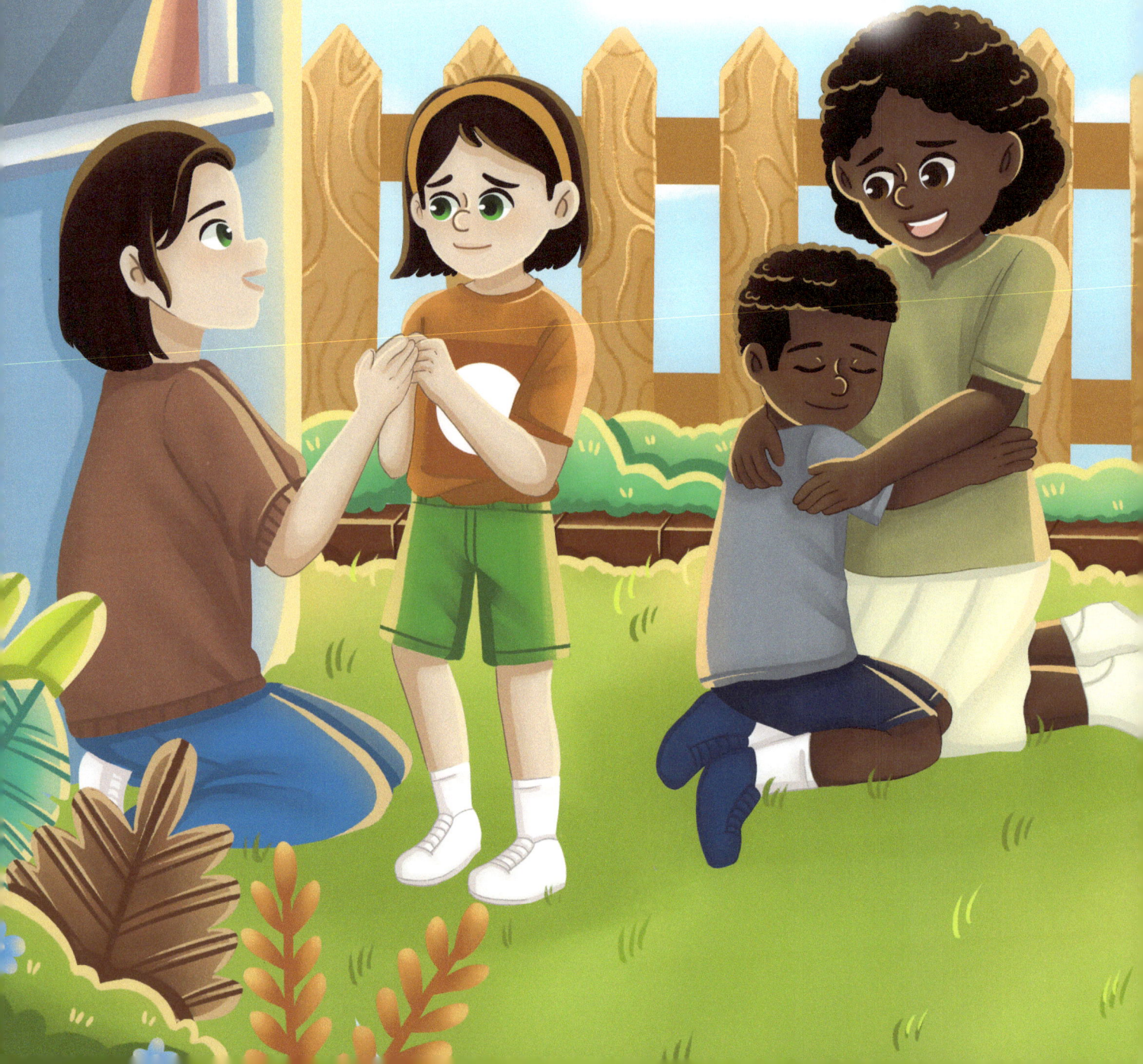

having these feelings,
is not something bad.

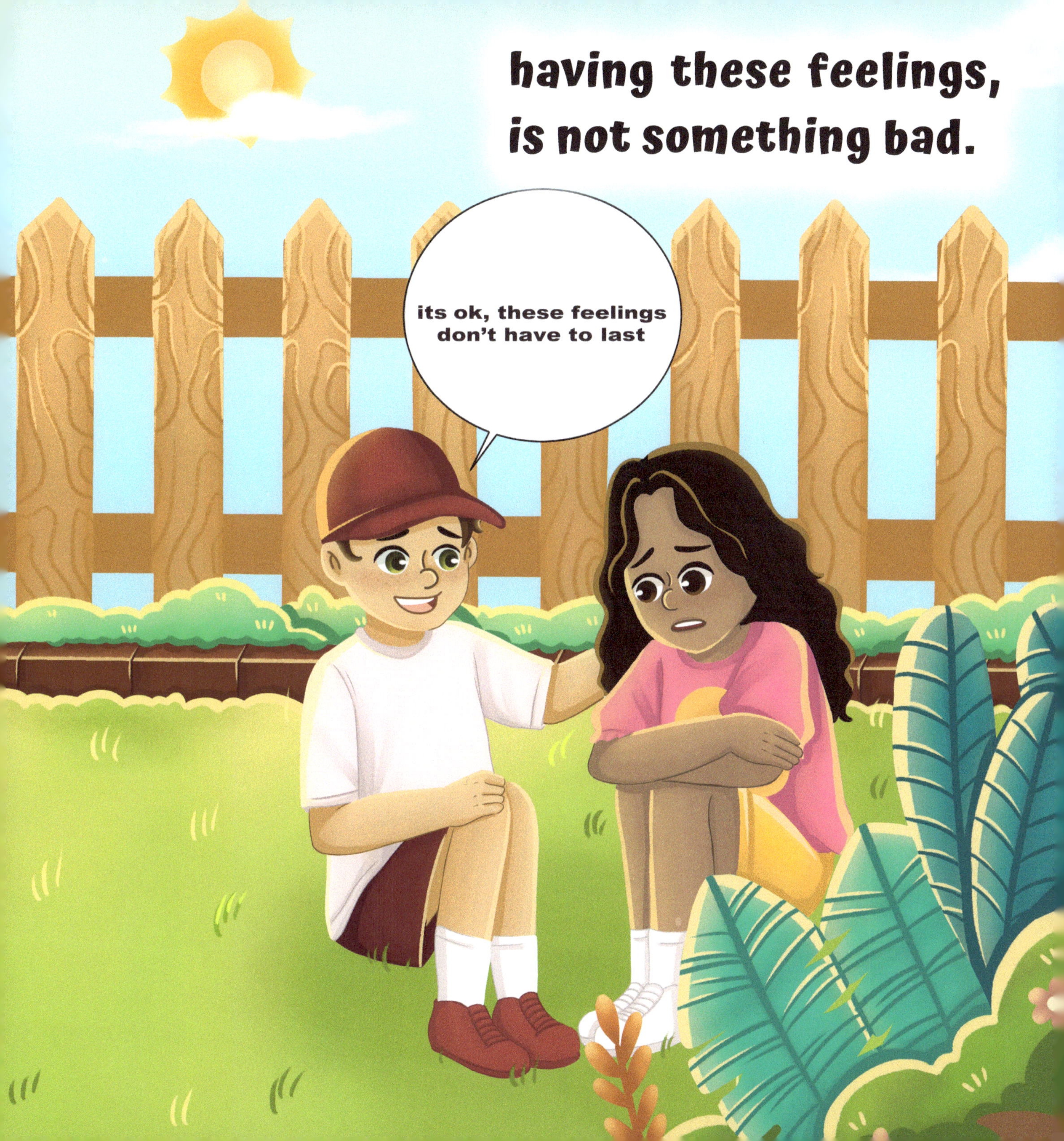

Take a deep
breath, nice
and slow,

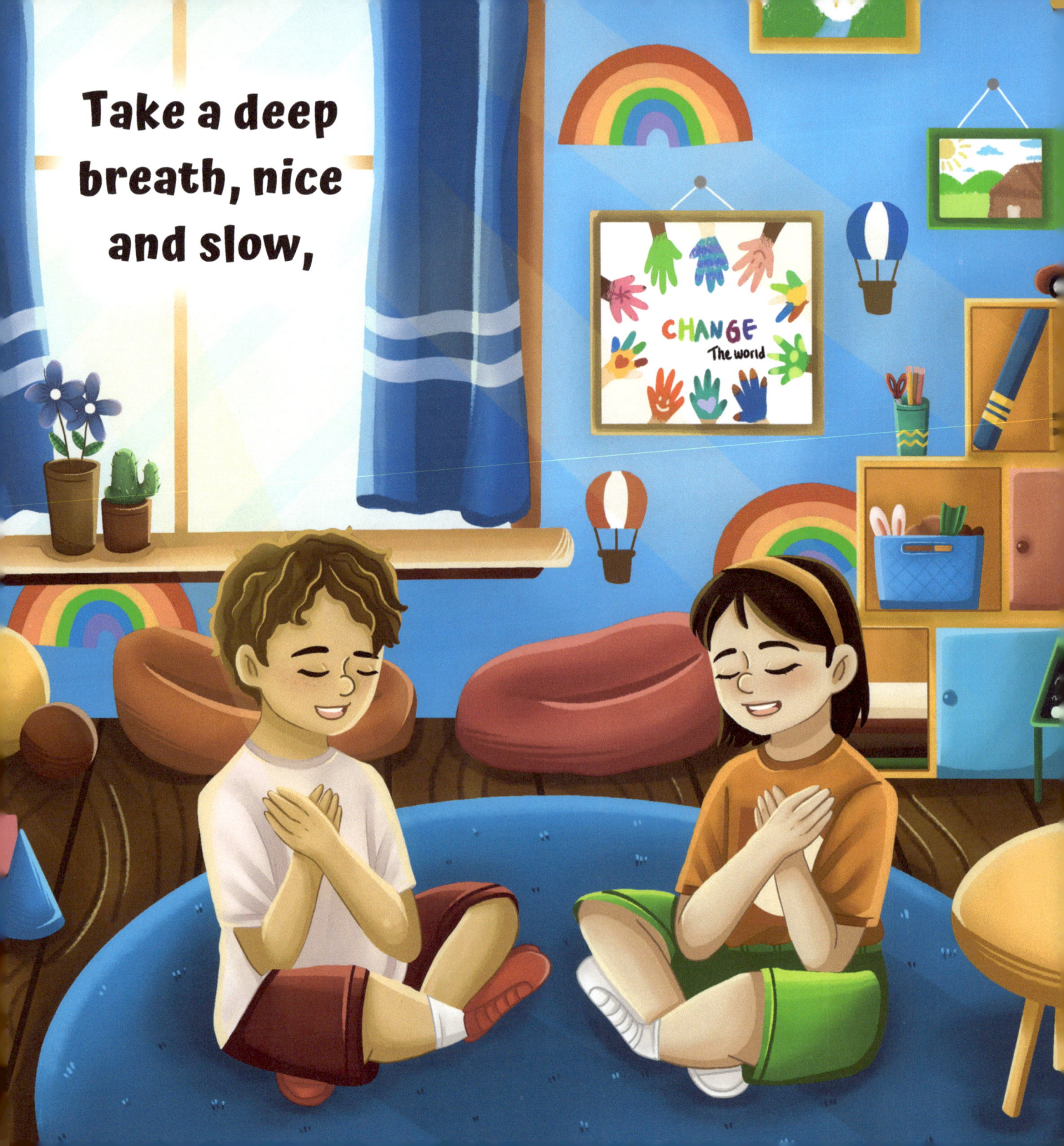

feel the air and
let worries go.

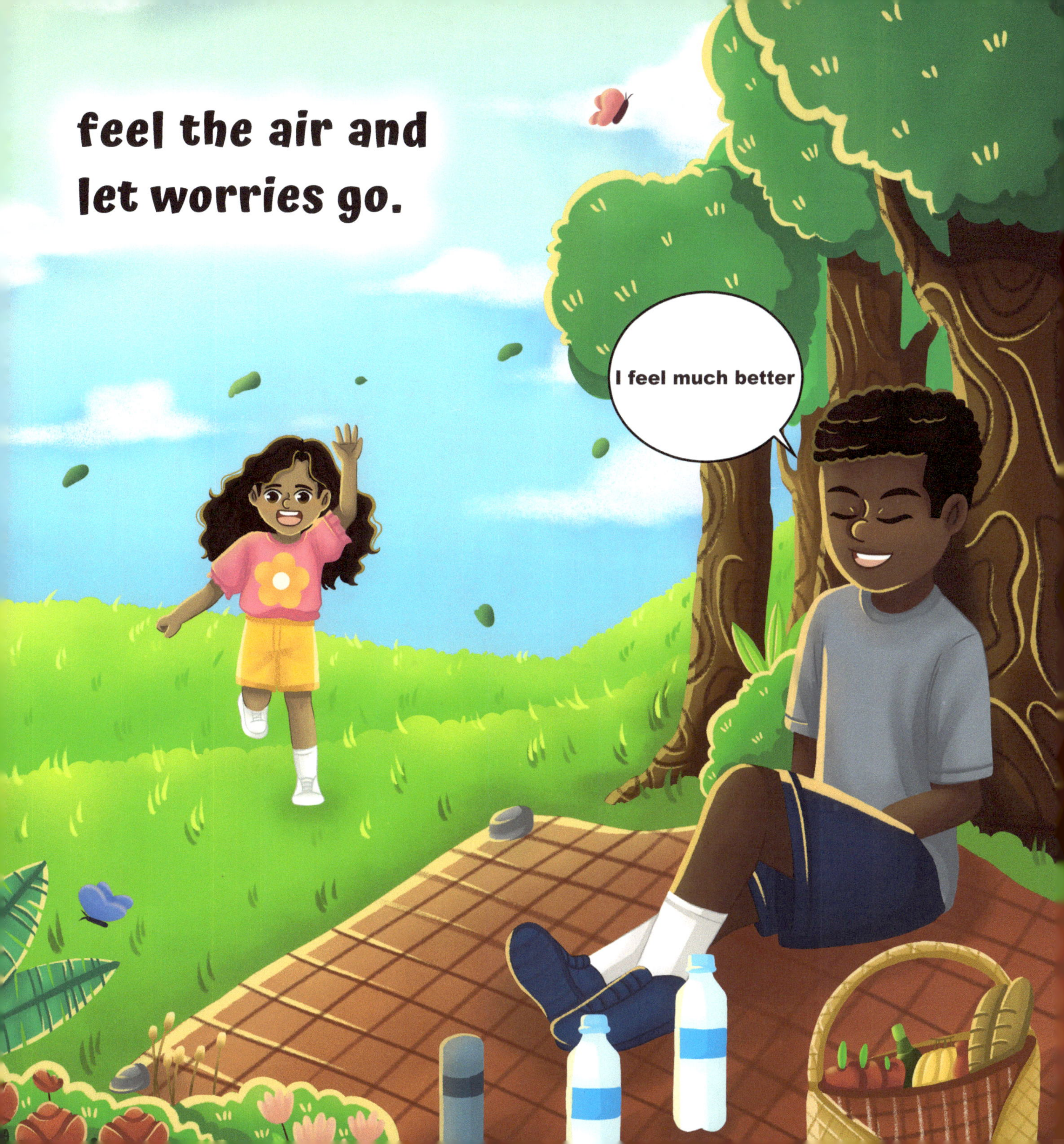

Take a break or count to 10,

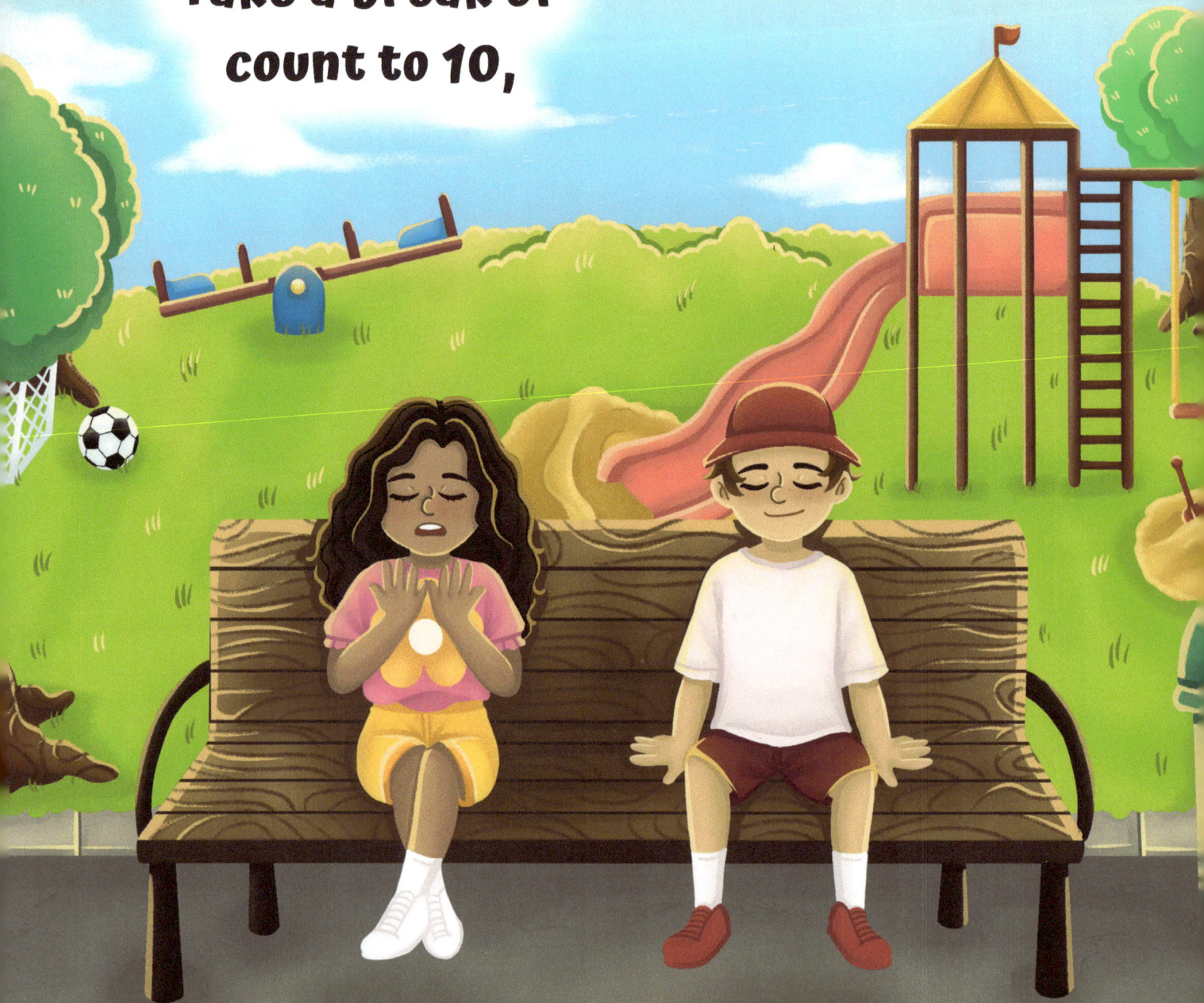

are ways we become calm
and start over again.

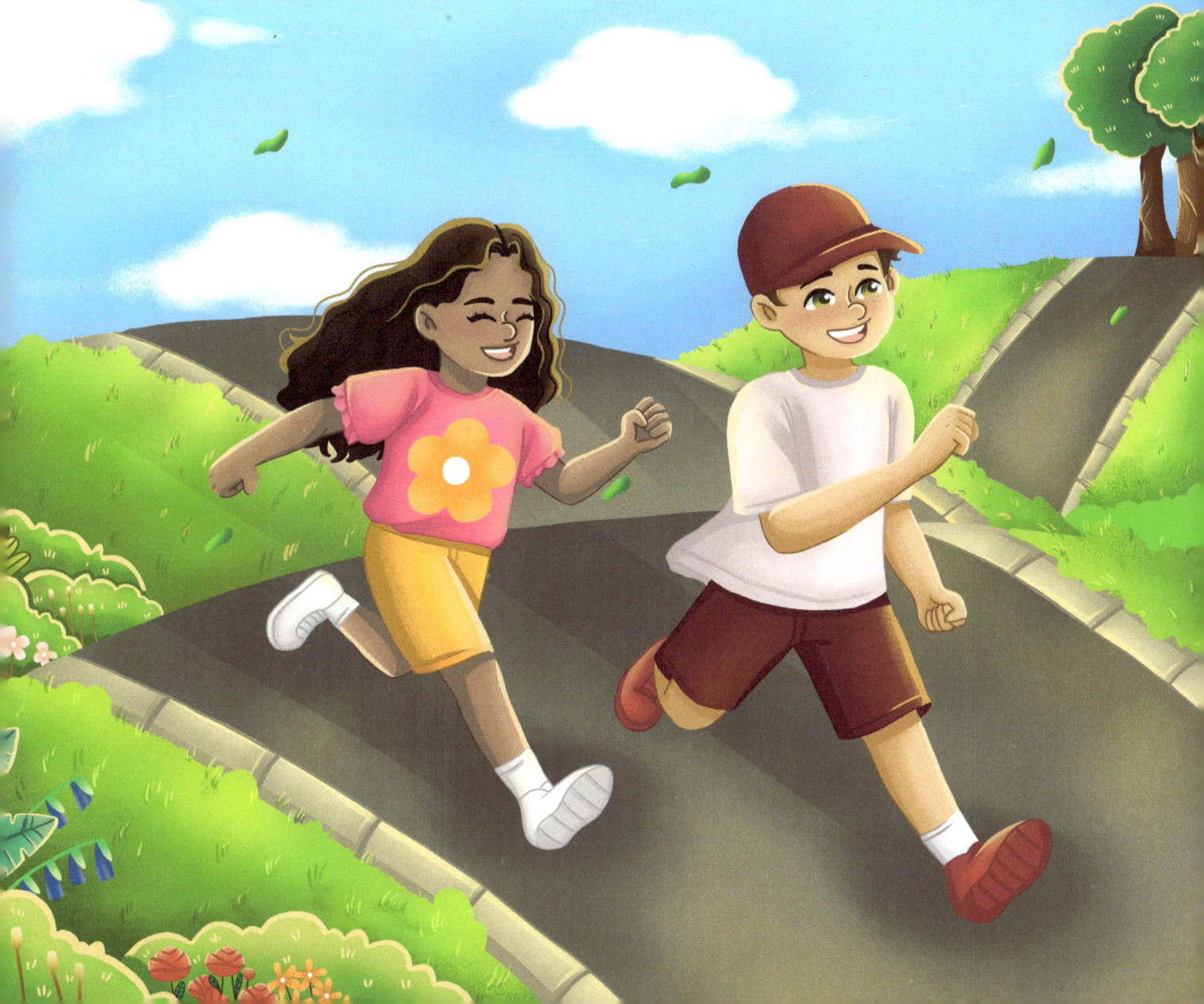

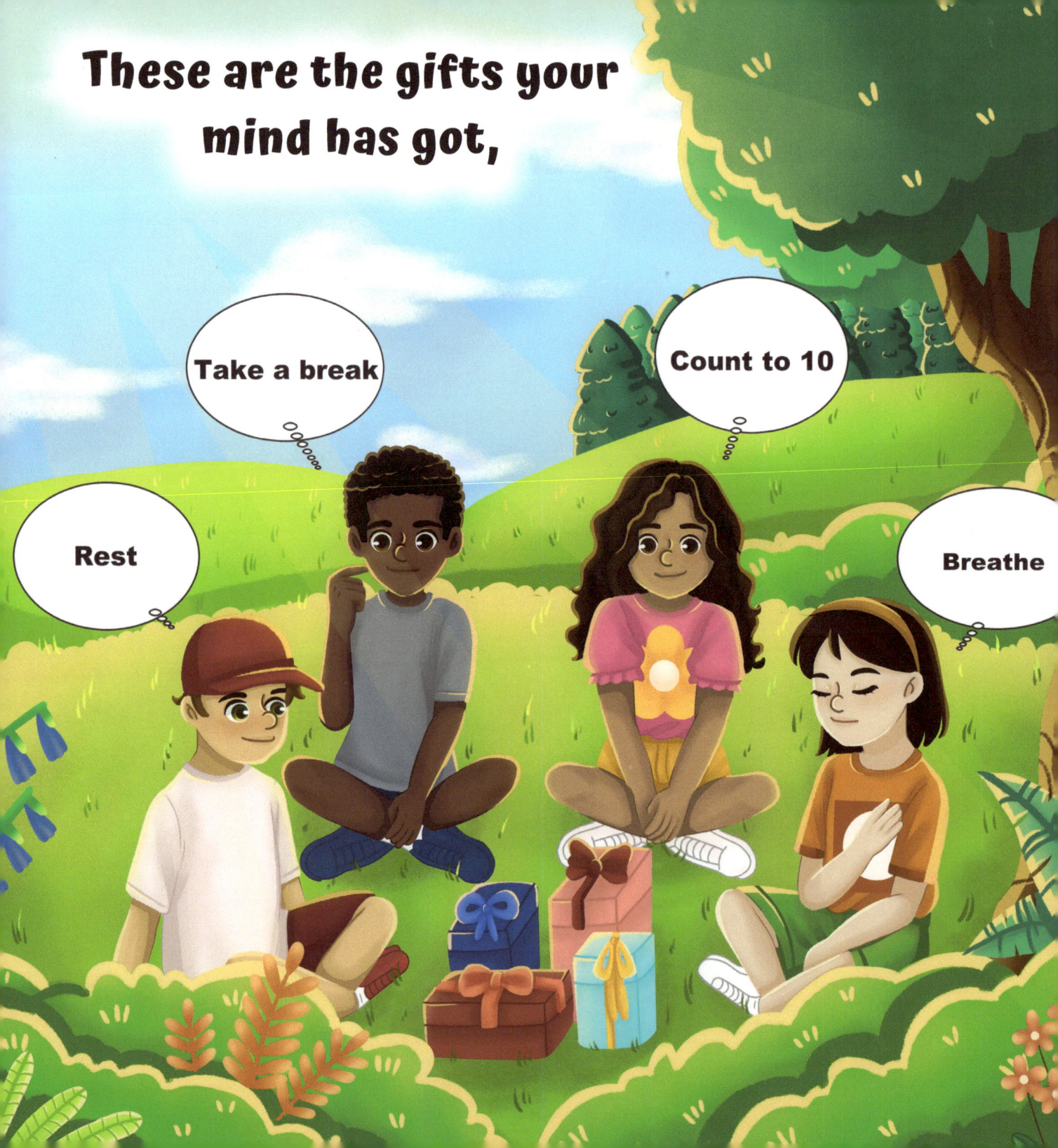

in every moment,
a thankful
thought.

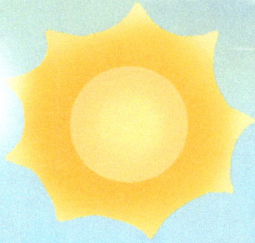

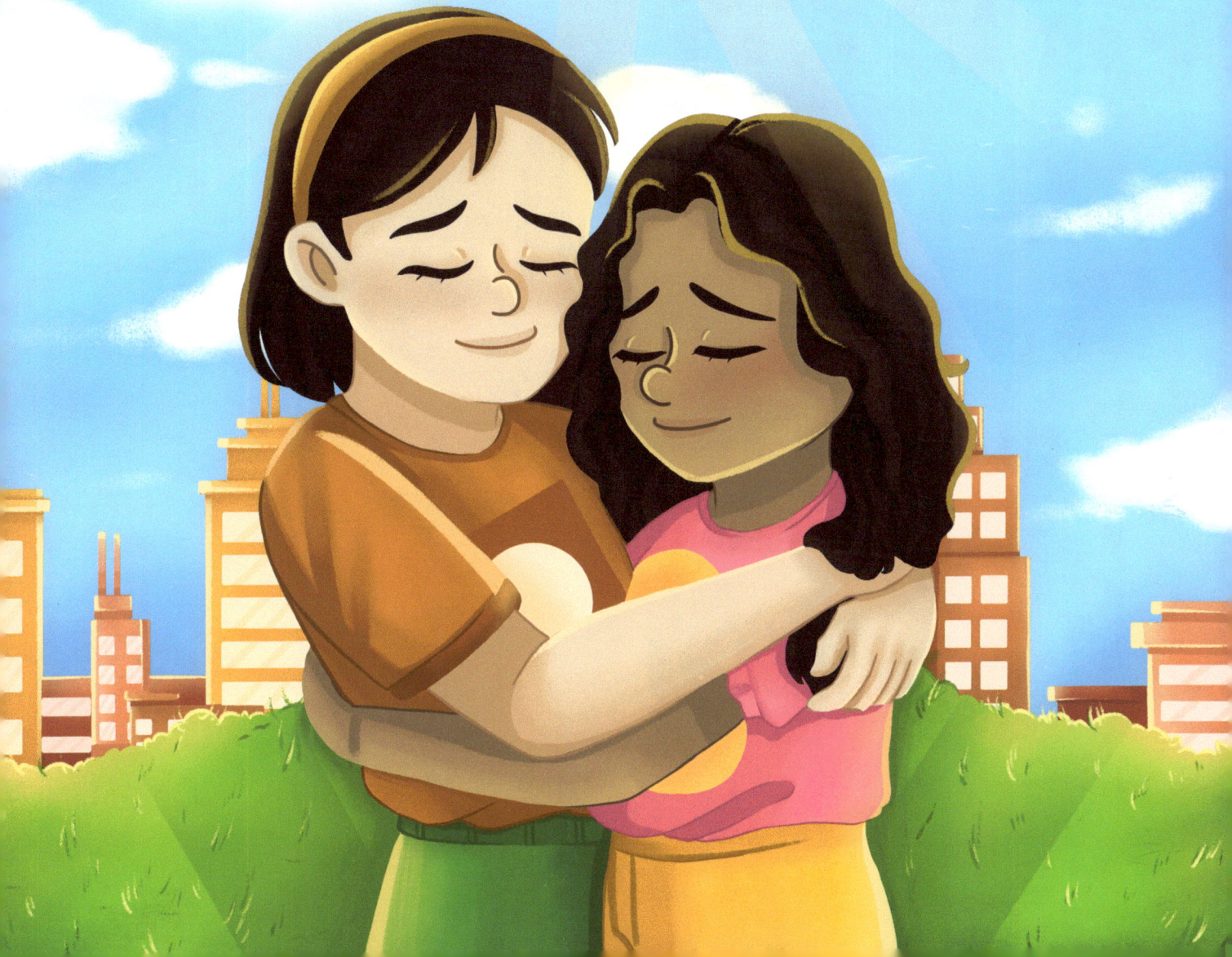

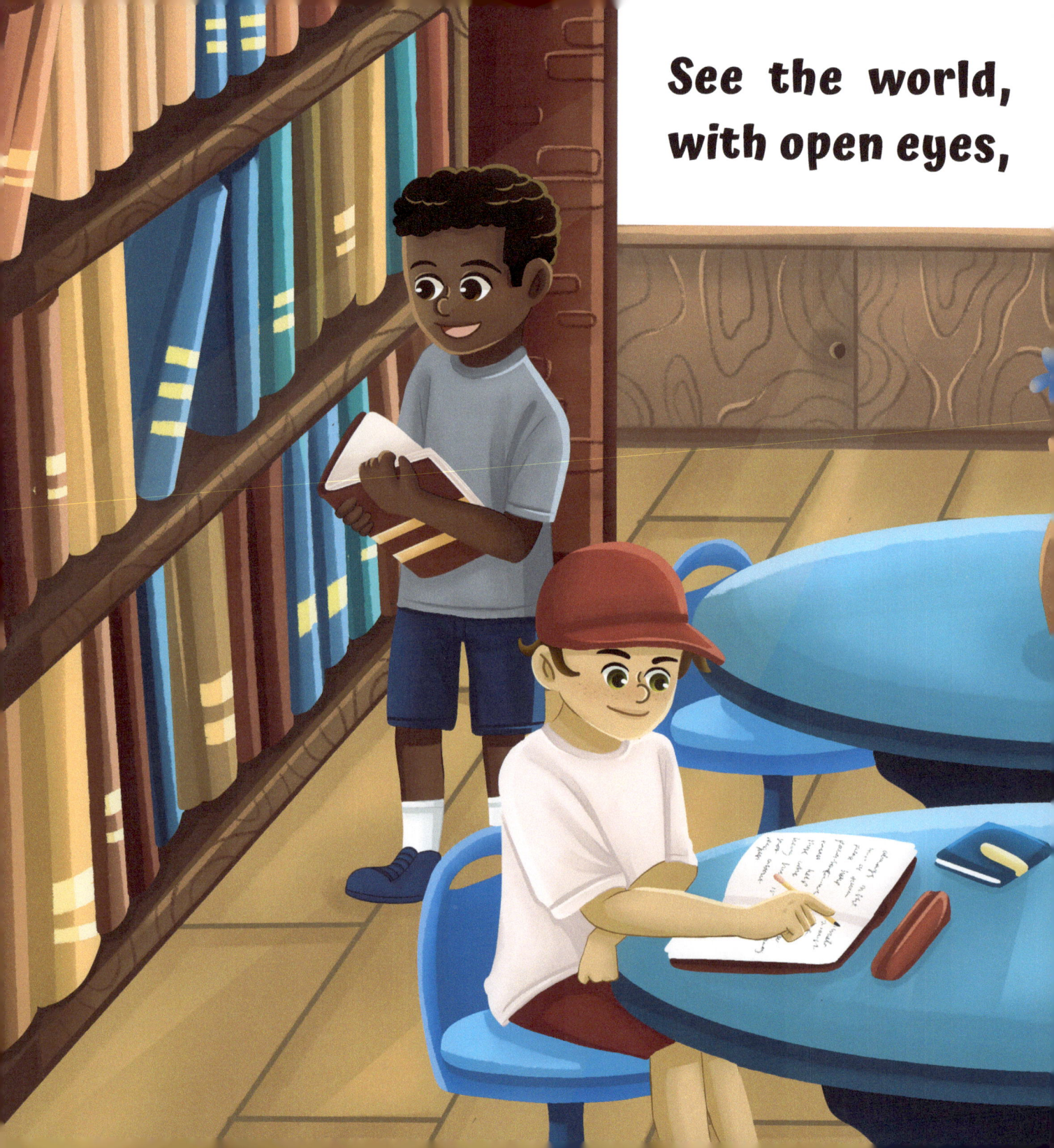

See the world,
with open eyes,

you are learning as you go and becoming so wise.

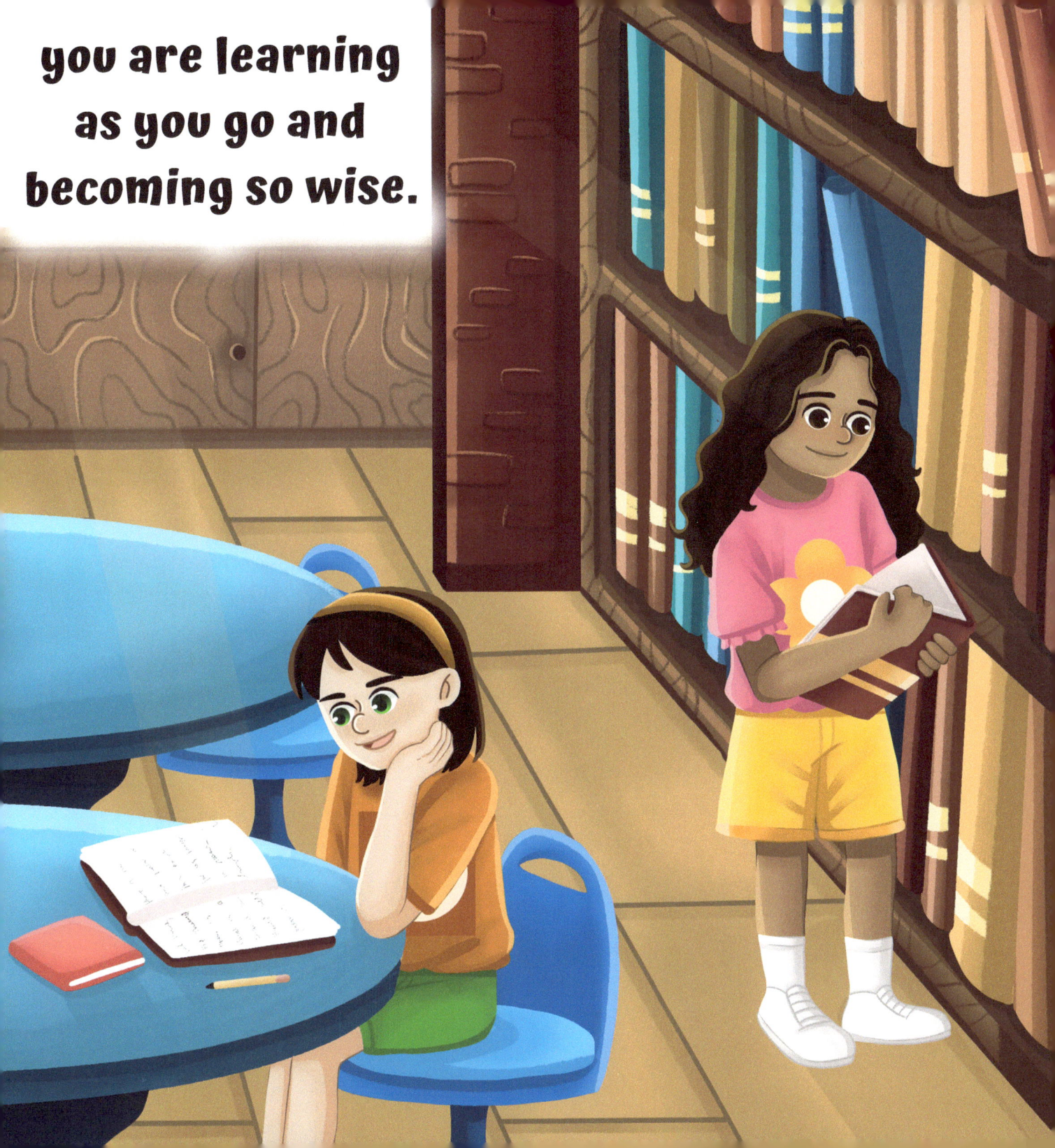

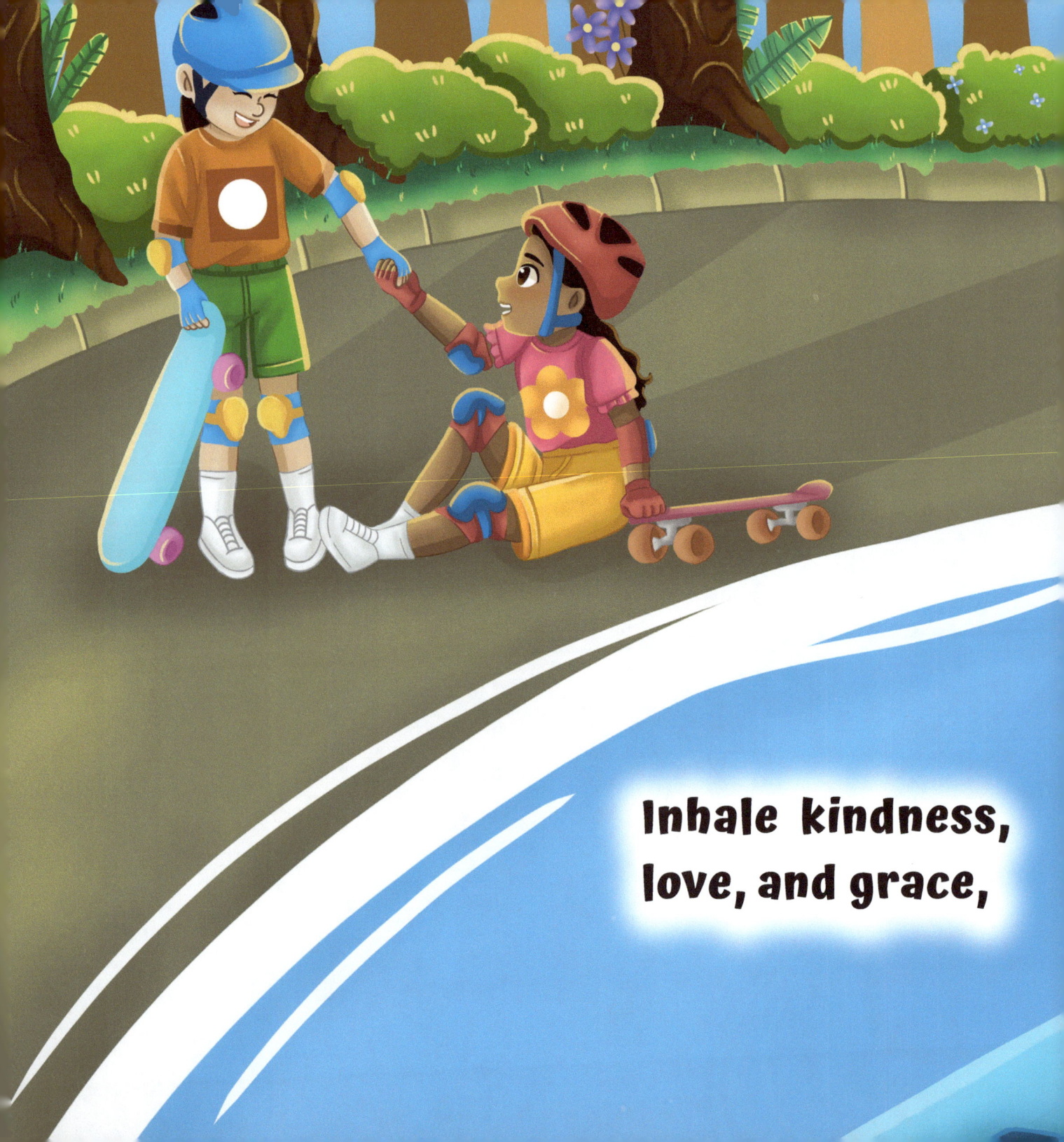

Inhale kindness,
love, and grace,

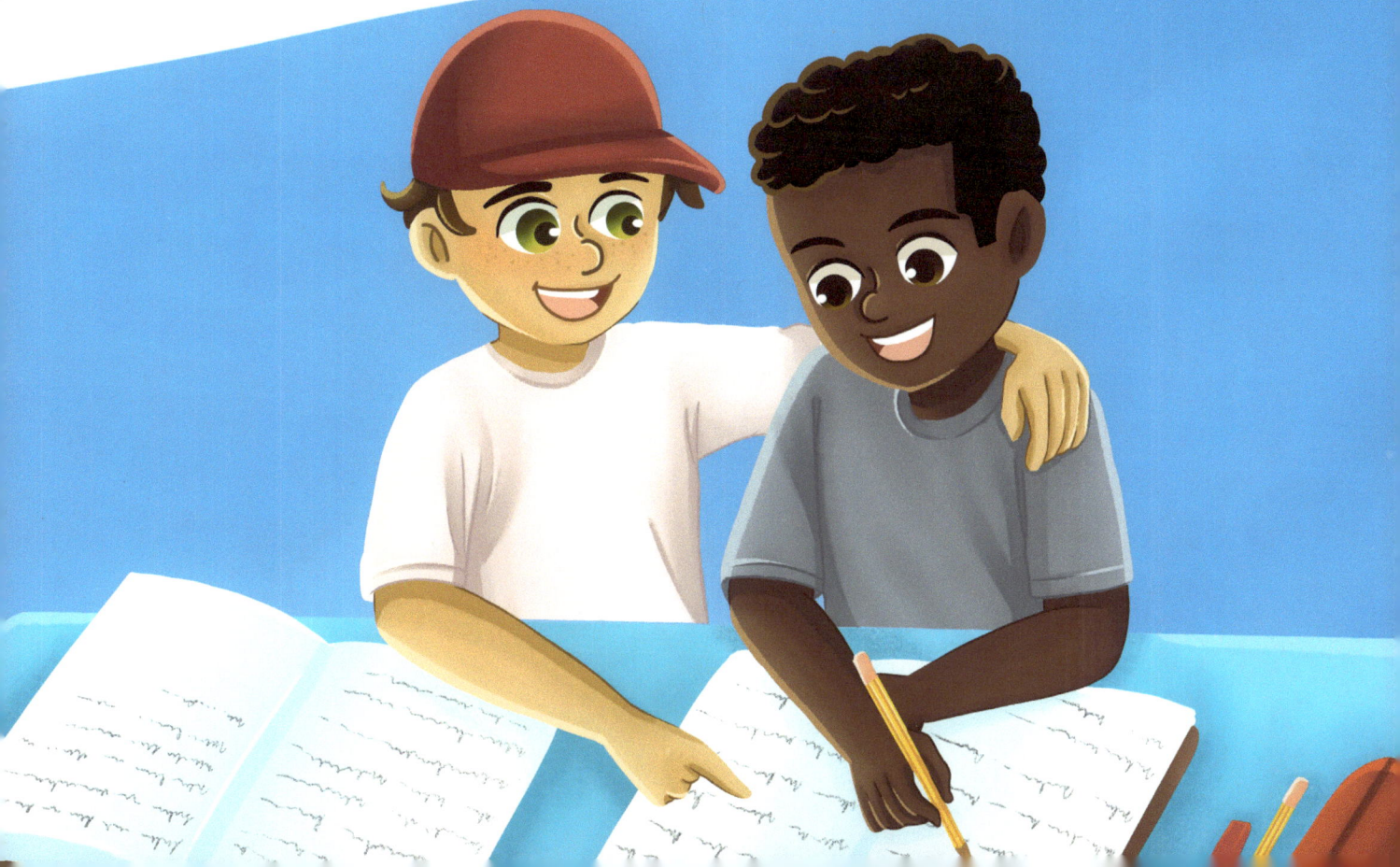

exhale worries, and
any fears we will face.

As day turns into starry night,

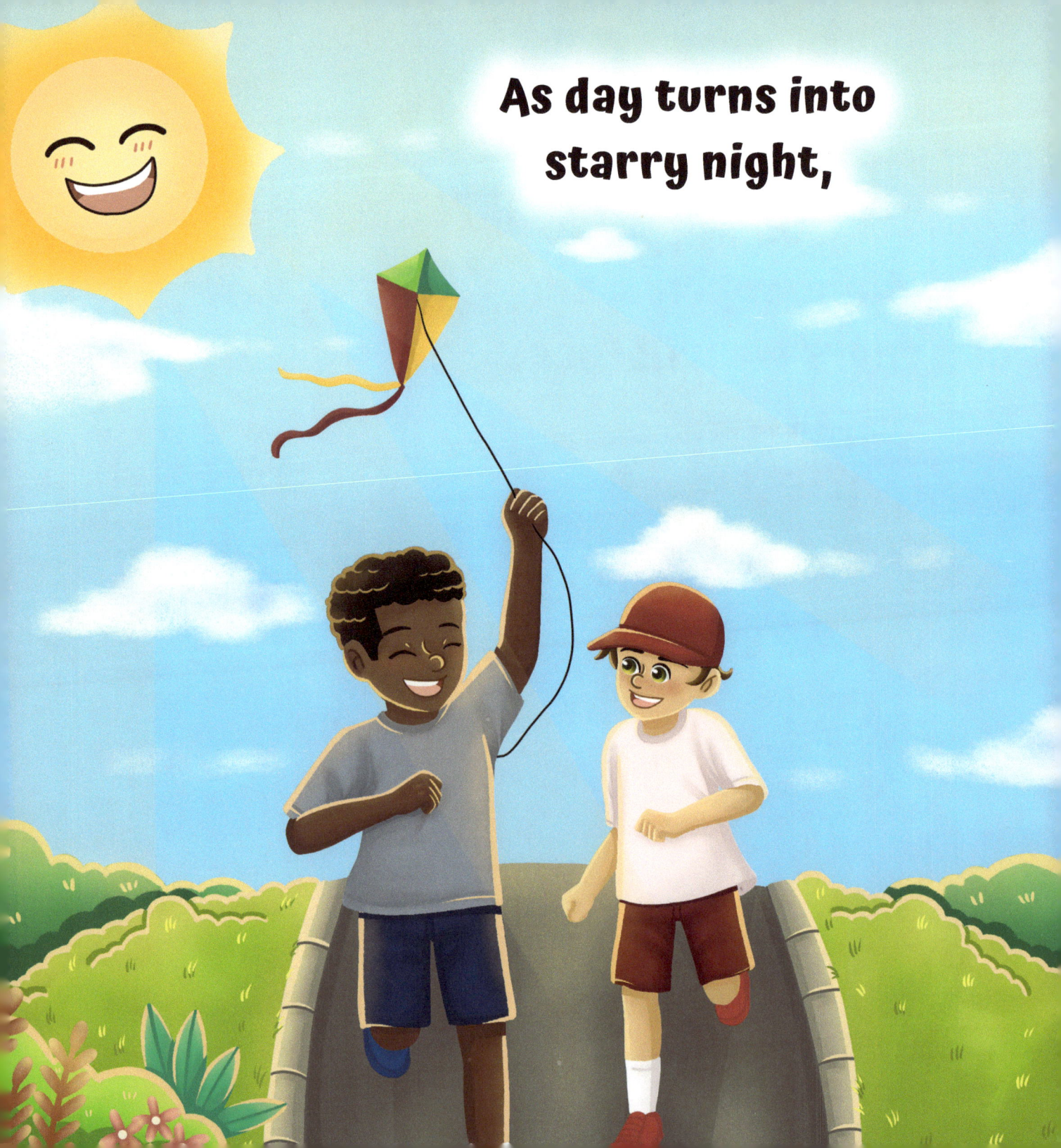

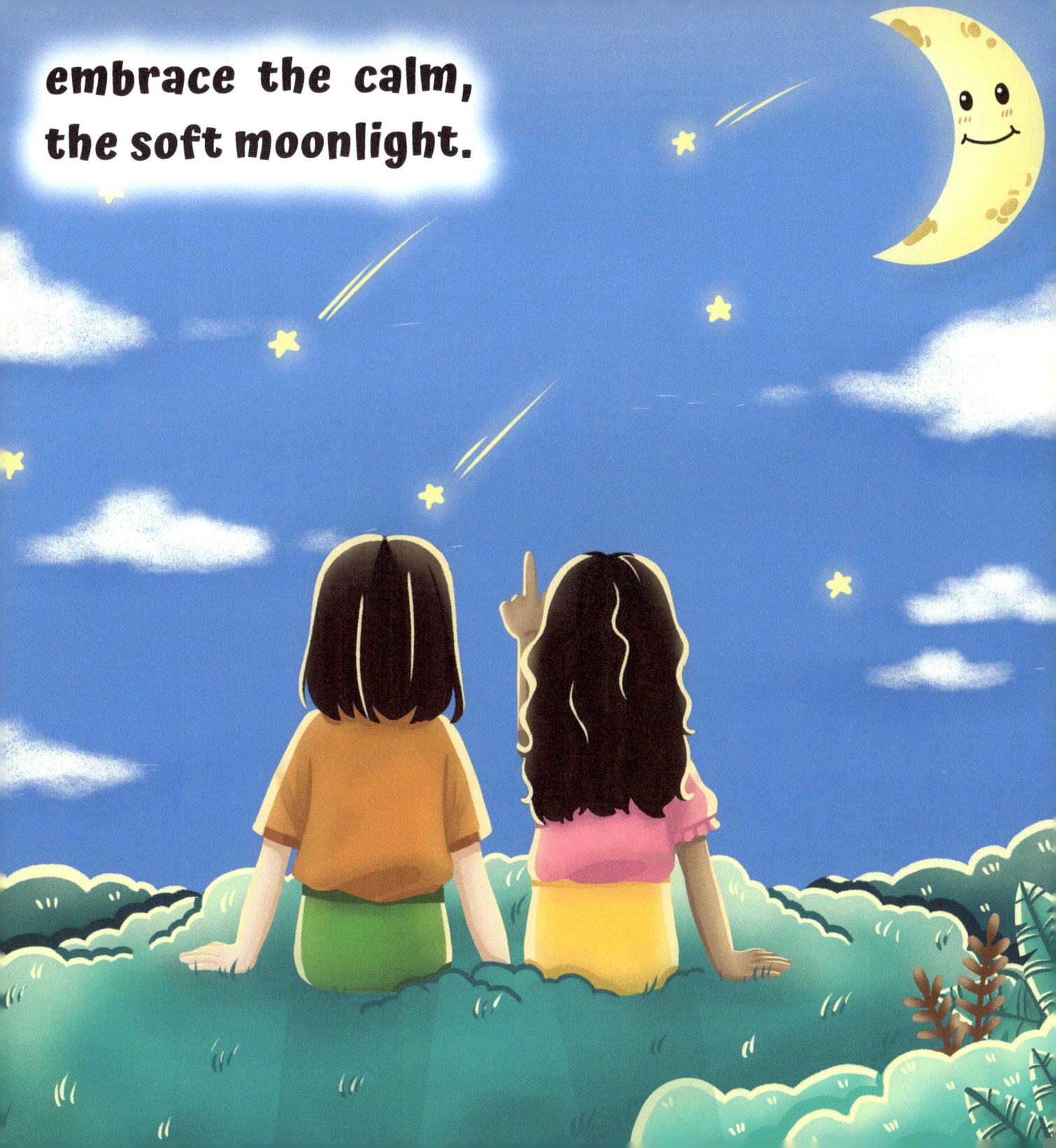

embrace the calm,
the soft moonlight.

Rest your mind and feel so free,

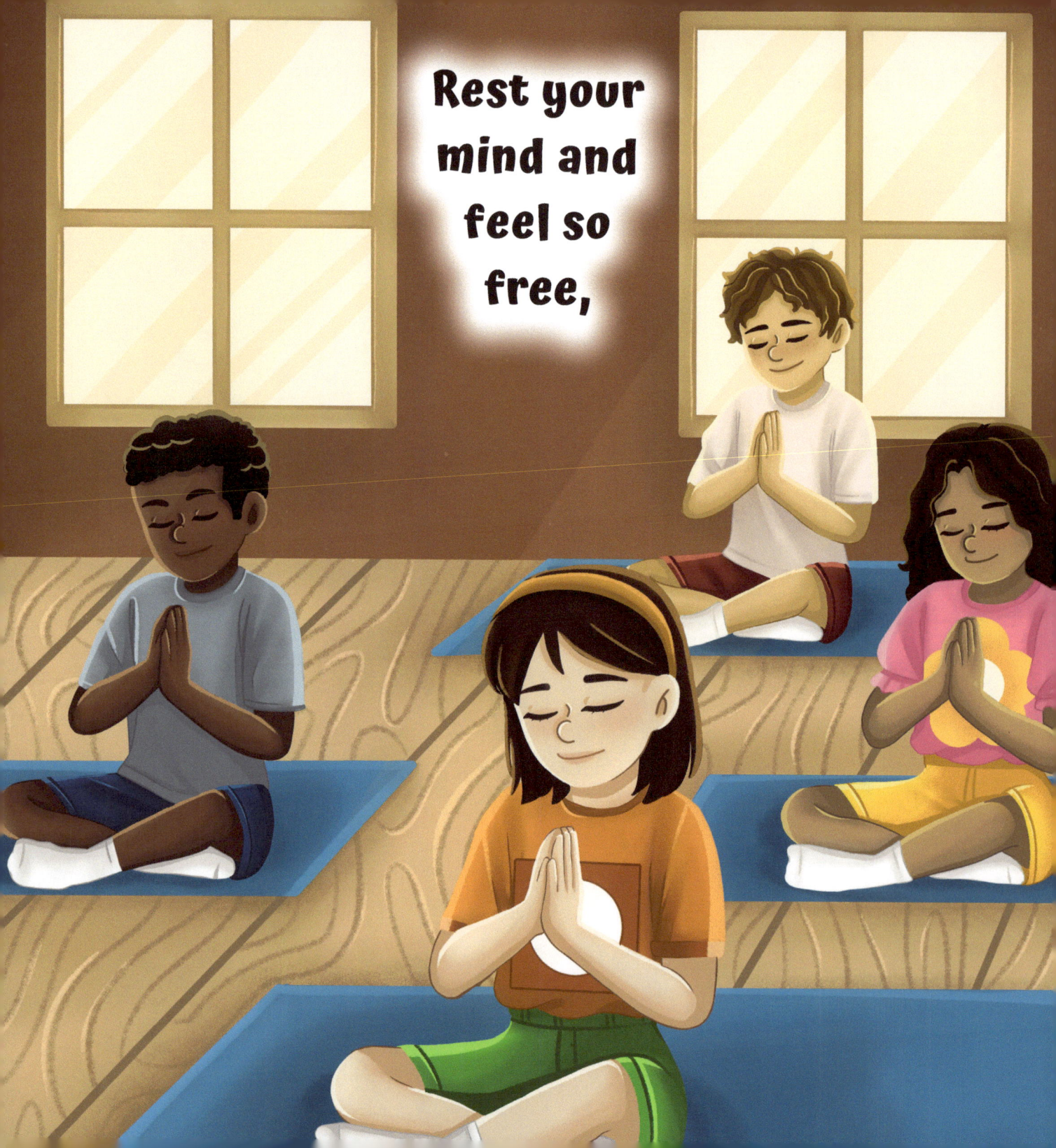

in dreams a Mindful Me, is what I will be.

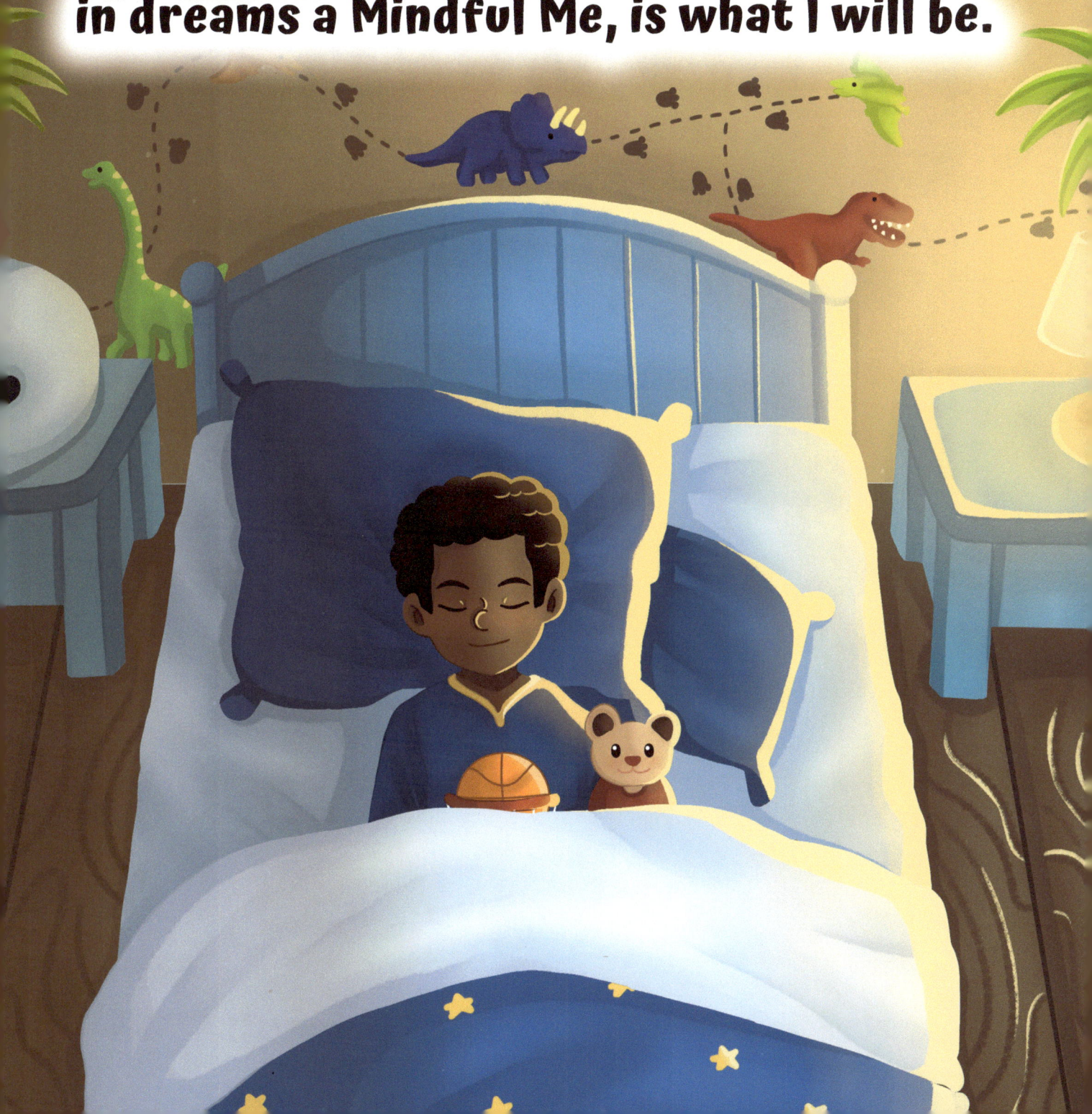

With every breath,
with every rhyme,

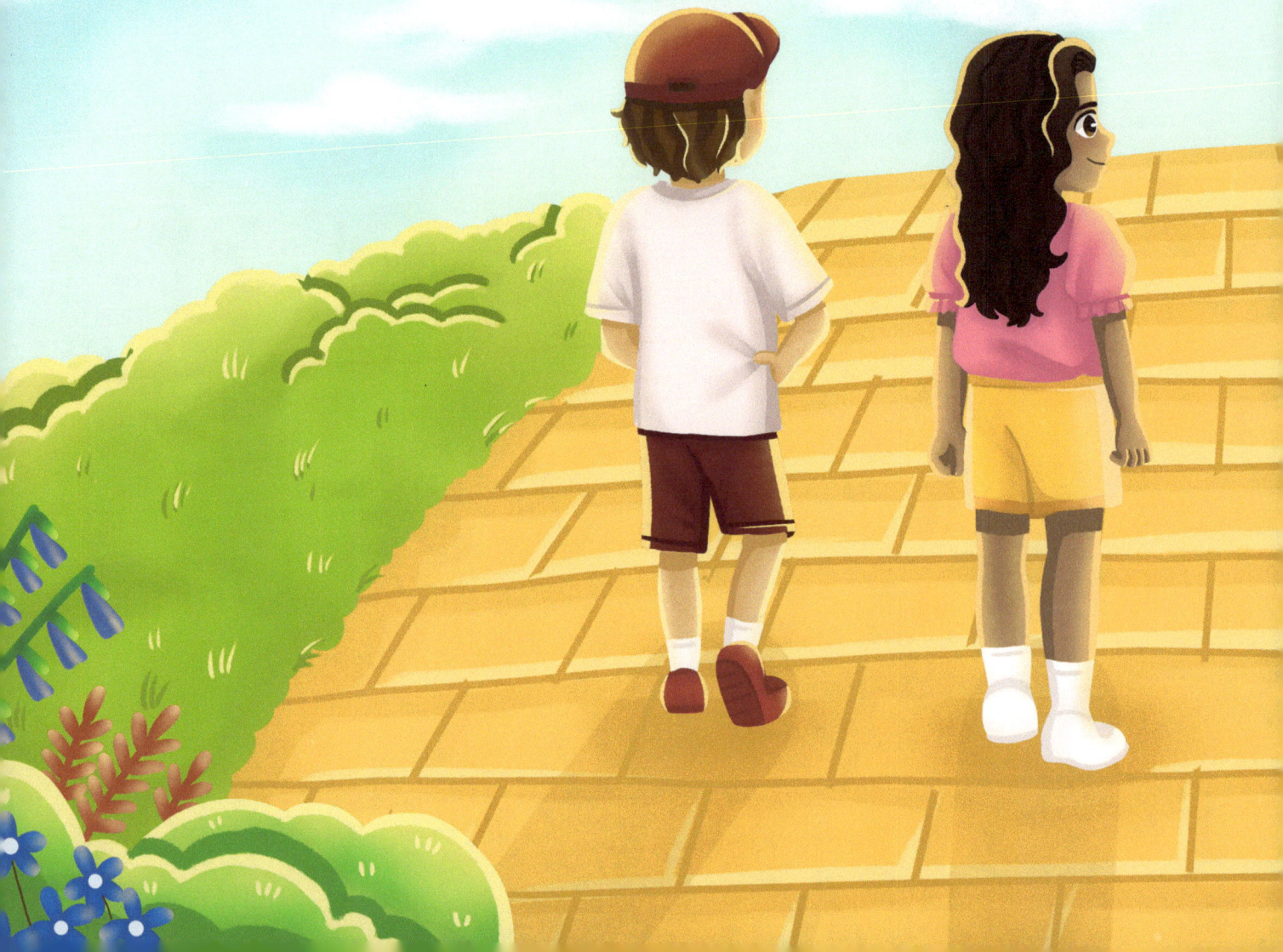

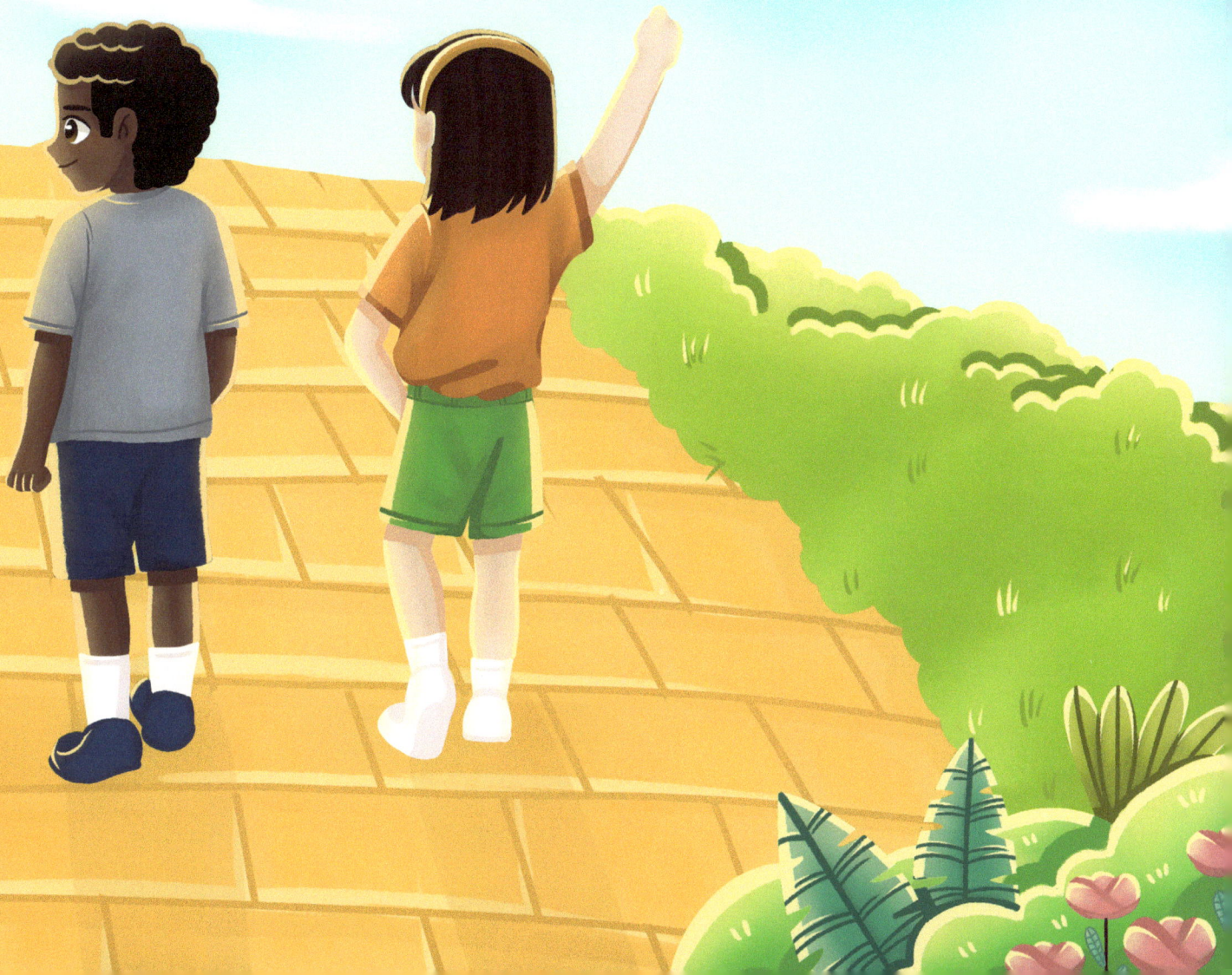

Mindful Me, until the end of time.

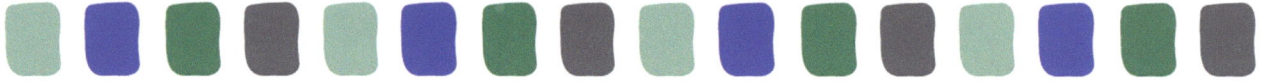

mind·ful·ness

noun

a mental state achieved by focusing one's awareness on the present moment, while calmly acknowledging and accepting one's feelings, thoughts and bodily sensations.

Studies have proven that mindfulness is effective. Children are not too young to learn to identify and label their wide range of emotions. Mindfulness is powerful for children to incorporate to navigate daily challenges and to help with feeling calm inside. With practice, mindfulness can also be an effective tool for staying in the present moment.

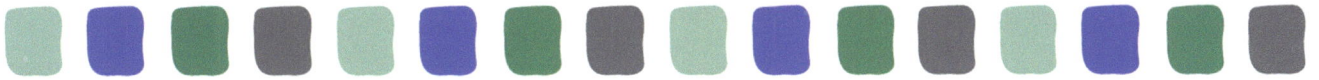

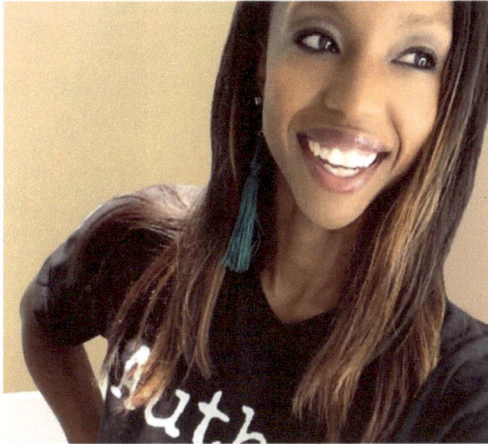

About The Author

Ashleigh is a mom of two and a Certified Empowerment Coach who teaches mindful strategies to her clients. Mindfulness became a very important part of her life – especially during the pandemic. During her own mindful routines, her children's curiosity often led them to jump in and do activities with her. Yoga and meditation are their favorites and they have incorporated kid versions to make it fun.

She hopes this book will motivate parents to encourage their children to practice mindfulness techniques. The mindful tools that are learned as children will lay the foundation to be utilized throughout their entire lives.

Stay connected for more from the Empower Books Collection.

: empowerbooks

empowerbooksforkids.net

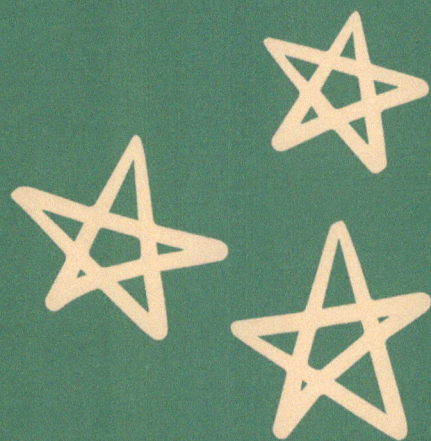